NEW FRONTIERS IN PSYCHOTROPIC DRUG RESEARCH

Edited by:

STUART FIELDING, Ph.D.

Associate Director of Biological Sciences
Manager of Pharmacology
Hoechst-Roussel Pharmaceuticals, Inc. Somerville New Jersey

and

RICHARD C. EFFLAND, Ph.D.

Associate Director of Chemical Research
Hoechst-Roussel Pharmaceuticals, Inc. Somerville New Jersey

FUTURA PUBLISHING COMPANY
Mount Kisco, New York
1979

Dedicated to Professor Dr. Rolf Sammet

Preface

This monograph is a result of a recent research seminar sponsored by Hoechst-Roussel Pharmaceuticals, Inc. When this seminar was planned, the first step was to stand back from the ongoing process of science to try to anticipate where the greatest activity might occur during the next decade. The participants were asked to predict the future, to determine the most promising lines of research, and to focus on those fields of psychopharmacology most likely to augment the activities of our own drug development program.

We are proud to present views of those scientists who are known to be experts in their fields, good of exposition, and open to multidisciplinary give and take. We are privileged to be the beneficiary of the thoughts of these scientists who accepted invitations to survey the state of their art, their major issues, their major hypotheses, and to state their major findings. The authors represented here need little introduction.

Dr. Joseph Schildkraut is the author of the catecholamine hypothesis of depression, a concept which has generated many years of fruitful research in the understanding of this disease. Dr. Arnold Friedhoff is the President of the American College of Neuropsychopharmacology and Dr. Fridolin Sulser is the President-elect of this prestigious organization which is considered by many to chart the future of neuropsychopharmacology research. Dr. Harbans Lal is known for contributions to many areas of drug development, among them are non-addicting drugs to treat opiate addicts, examining the chronic effects of neuroleptics, and the development of new antidiarrheals, just to name a few. His novel technique of drug discrimination is now being used in many pharmaceutical companies to screen new drugs of different categories. Dr. Thomas Ban, a pioneer of clinical psychopharmacology, has devoted many fruitful years to geropsychiatry and with his help has become a rapidly emerging corallary to the field of drug development. Dr. Arthur J. Prange, Jr., is known for studying the effects of peptides in mental illness. The research that has been started by him is now being carried out in many laboratories throughout the world. Dr. George U. Balis has opened up various areas of study in episodic dyscontrol behavior. The effects of drugs on this behavior is now beginning to show fruitful results and we can expect selective compounds to be developed some time in the near future. And finally, Dr. Calvin Reed Brown, Medical Director at Utah State Prison, who has uncovered parodoxical rage reactions produced by benzodiazepines in the prison population.

Needless to say, the topics selected to be included in this monograph are not meant to cover all areas of research but rather to emphasize a few areas as cases in point. We hope that this series can be continued to cover many areas of psychotropic drug development in the future.

Stuart Fielding, Ph.D.
Richard C. Effland, Ph.D.

Contributors

George U. Balis, M.D.
Professor of Psychiatry
Institute of Psychiatry and Human Behavior
University of Maryland
School of Medicine
Baltimore, Maryland

Thomas A. Ban, M.D.
Professor of Psychiatry
Vanderbilt University
Nashville, Tennessee

Calvin Reed Brown, M.D.
Medical Director
Utah State Prison
Draper, Utah

Jonathan O. Cole, M.D.
Lecturer in Psychiatry
Harvard Medical School
Boston, Massachusetts
Head, Psychopharmacology Dept.
McLean Hospital
Belmont, Massachusetts

Arnold J. Friedhoff, M.D.
Millhauser Laboratories
Department of Psychiatry
New York University Medical Center
New York, New York

Jon E. Gudeman, M.D.
Associate Professor of Psychiatry
Harvard Medical School
Director of Adult Services
Massachusetts Mental Health Center
Boston, Massachusetts

James M. Herzog, M.D.
Instructor of Psychiatry
Harvard Medical School
Staff Physician
Childrens Hospital Medical Center
Boston, Massachusetts

Richard A. LaBrie, M.D.
Statistical Consultant
LaBrie Associates
Cambridge, Massachusetts

Harbans Lal, Ph.D.
Professor of Pharmacology, Toxicology and Psychology
University of Rhode Island
Kingston, Rhode Island

Peter T. Loosen, M.D.
Biological Sciences Research Center
Department of Psychiatry
University of North Carolina
School of Medicine
Chapel Hill, North Carolina

Kalidas Nandy, M.D., Ph.D.
Associate Director
Grecc Veterans Administration Hospital
Bedford, Massachusetts

Charles B. Nemeroff, Ph.D.
Biological Sciences Research Center
Department of Psychiatry
University of North Carolina
School of Medicine
Chapel Hill, North Carolina

Paul J. Orsulak, Ph.D.
Assistant Professor of Psychiatry
Harvard Medical School
Boston, Massachusetts

Arthur J. Prange, Jr., M.D.
Biological Sciences Research Center
Department of Psychiatry
University of North Carolina
School of Medicine
Chapel Hill, North Carolina

William A. Rohde, M.D.
Clinical Instructor
Harvard Medical School
Boston, Massachusetts
Assistant Attending Psychiatrist
McLean Hospital
Belmont, Massachusetts

Allan F. Schatzberg, M.D.
Assistant Professor of Psychiatry
Harvard Medical School
Boston, Massachusetts
Associate Psychiatrist
McLean Hospital
Belmont, Massachusetts

Joseph J. Schildkraut, M.D.
Department of Psychiatry
Harvard Medical School
Neuropsychopharmacology Laboratory
Massachusetts Mental Health Center
Boston, Massachusetts
McLean Hospital
Belmont, Massachusetts

Fridolin Sulser, M.D.
Vanderbilt University
School of Medicine
Tennessee Neuropsychiatric Institute
Nashville, Tennessee

Acknowledgment

Although it is impossible to cite the valuable assistance given to us by many people at Hoechst-Roussel Pharmaceuticals, Inc., the helpful suggestions, encouragement, and critical decision making provided by Dr. Grover C. Helsley, Vice President of Research, is especially appreciated.

Contents

1

Biochemical Discrimination of Subgroups of Affective and Schizophrenic Disorders

JOSEPH J. SCHILDKRAUT, M.D., PAUL J. ORSULAK, PH.D., ALAN F. SCHATZBERG, M.D., JAMES M. HERZOG, M.D., JON E. GUDEMAN, M.D., JONATHAN O. COLE, M.D., WILLIAM A. ROHDE, M.D. and RICHARD A. LaBRIE, PH.D.

I. INTRODUCTION

The possibility that depressive disorders might be divided into subgroups characterized by differences in catecholamine metabolism was first raised over ten years ago (43); but it is only in more recent years that we have begun to see the emergence of data consistent with this possibility. In this paper, we shall briefly summarize aspects of our recent research findings suggesting that we can discriminate three biochemically discrete subgroups of depressive disorders on the basis of measurements of urinary catecholamines and metabolites as well as platelet monoamine oxidase (MAO) activity. Moreover, we shall also summarize aspects of our studies showing differences in platelet MAO activity among subgroups of schizophrenic disorders. The methods used in these studies, as well as the findings summarized in this paper, have been reported in greater detail elsewhere (52, 50, 37).

II. BIOCHEMICAL DISCRIMINATION OF SUBGROUPS OF AFFECTIVE DISORDERS

A number of lines of evidence now suggest that 3-methoxy-4-hydroxyphenylglycol (MHPG) is the major metabolite of norepinephrine in human brain as it is in the brains of a number of other

This work was supported in part by Grant No. MH15413 from the National Institute of Mental Health and by a grant from the Scottish Rite Schizophrenia Research Program, N.M.J., USA.

Psychotropic Drug Research

species (41, 42, 31, 18, 40, 27, 29, 60).* Urinary MHPG also may derive, in part, from the peripheral sympathetic nervous system as well as from the brain (41, 2), and the exact fraction of urinary MHPG which does, in fact, derive from norepinephrine originating in the brain remains uncertain (29, 8, 22, 23, 14). However, recent findings suggest that, in man, the contribution from brain may be greater than 50% (26).

In our initial longitudinal studies of individual patients with naturally occurring or amphetamine-induced bipolar manic-depressive episodes, we found that levels of urinary MHPG were relatively lower during depressions and higher during manic or hypomanic episodes than during periods of remission (20, 49, 53, 58); and these findings have now been confirmed by a number of other investigators (6, 7, 12, 38, 35), though all findings do not concur (10, 55).

However, all depressions are not clinically or biologically homogenous (43), and all depressed patients do not excrete comparably low levels of MHPG (30). Thus, our research next explored the possibility that the urinary excretion of MHPG and other catecholamine metabolites might provide a biochemical basis for differentiating among the depressive disorders. As shown in Table I, in our initial study, we found that MHPG excretion was significantly lower in a small group of patients with bipolar manic-depressive depressions than in patients with unipolar nonendogenous chronic characterological depressions (47, 48); and these differences in

TABLE I

Differences in urinary MHPG levels in patients with
bipolar manic-depressive and unipolar nonendogenous
(chronic characterological) depressions.

Subtype of Depression	N	MHPG Level ($\mu g/24\,hr$)
Bipolar Manic-Depressive	5	1240 ± 160†
Unipolar Nonendogenous (Chronic Characterological)	5	1800 ± 90†

Data are expressed as means ± standard errors of the means.
†$p < 0.02$ for difference between bipolar manic-depressive and unipolar nonendogenous depressions.

*In contrast, relatively little urinary norepinephrine, normetanephrine, epinephrine, metanephrine, and 3-methoxy-4-hydroxymandelic acid (VMA) appear to derive from the central nervous system, and most is thought to originate in peripheral sources, i.e., the sympathetic nervous system or the adrenal gland.

2

MHPG excretion in depressed patients could not be accounted for by differences in retardation, agitation, or anxiety (44). Our findings of reduced MHPG excretion in bipolar manic-depressive depressions have now been confirmed by other investigators (19, 28, 17), and in our more recent studies we have extended these findings.

The urinary excretion of MHPG has now been measured in a series of 63 depressed patients studied under drug-free conditions. As shown in Figure 1, when compared with values observed in patients with unipolar nonendogenous depressions (the principal comparison group used in this study) or in patients with unipolar endogenous depressions (characterized by specific research criteria), we found reduced mean levels of urinary MHPG in patients with schizophrenia-related depressions (characterized by histories of

MHPG EXCRETION IN SUBTYPES OF DEPRESSIVE DISORDERS

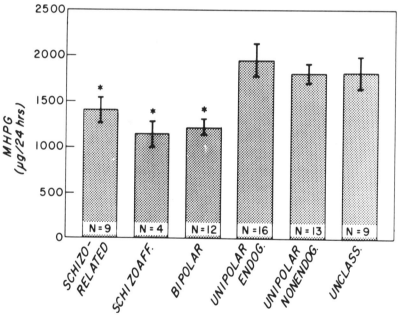

FIGURE 1   MHPG excretion in subtypes of depressive disorders. MHPG was determined in two to ten separate 24-hour urine samples obtained from each patient, and the average value for each patient was plotted. This study included patients with the following subtypes of depressive disorders: schizophrenia-related (N=9), schizoaffective (N=4), bipolar manic-depressive (N=12), unipolar endogenous (N=16), unipolar nonendogenous (N=13), and unclassifiable (N=9).

Psychotropic Drug Research

chronic asocial behavior), in patients with schizoaffective depressions (characterized by affect nonconsonant delusions or hallucinations occurring in the absence of a history of chronic asocial behavior), and in patients with bipolar manic-depressive depressions (characterized by a prior history of mania requiring some form of clinical intervention).* There were no significant differences among these groups in Hamilton Depression Rating Scale scores (21), urine volume, or creatinine excretion.

The distribution of MHPG values below and above 1500 micrograms per day was compared in these clinically defined subtypes of depressive disorders. As shown in Table II, 14 of the 16 patients with bipolar manic-depressive or schizoaffective depressions had MHPG levels less than 1500 micrograms per day, whereas 12 of the 13 patients with unipolar nonendogenous depressions had levels of MHPG that were greater than 1500 micrograms per day. The unipolar endogenous depressions were more biochemically heterogeneous, with 5 patients having MHPG levels less than 1500 micrograms per day while 11 patients had MHPG levels greater than 1500 micrograms per day.

We also measured the urinary excretion of norepinephrine, normetanephrine, epinephrine, metanephrine, and VMA in this study. As shown in Table III, the urinary excretion of norepinephrine tended to be low both in schizoaffective and in bipolar manic-depressive depressions. However, the differences between these groups and the unipolar nonendogenous depressions were only of borderline statistical significance. There were no other meaningful differences in norepinephrine or normetanephrine excretion in these various subtypes of depressive disorders.

As shown in Table IV, levels of urinary epinephrine and metanephrine were found to be significantly lower in schizophrenia-related depressions than in the unipolar nonendogenous depressions, or in any other of the subtypes of depressive disorders that we studied. This reduction in epinephrine and metanephrine excretion in schizophrenia-related depressions was unexpected and suggested the possibility that this might represent a discrete biochemical subgroup.

As shown in Table V, there were no meaningful differences in VMA excretion when values were compared in the various subtypes of depressive disorders. In contrast, recapitulating the data shown in Figure 1, MHPG excretion was significantly reduced in the

*The system we use for classifying depressive disorders has been described elsewhere (52).

4

TABLE II
Distribution of MHPG values
in subtypes of depressive disorders

MHPG (μg/24 hrs)	Schizo-Relat.	Schizo-aff.	Bipolar Manic-Dep.	Uni. Endog.	Uni. Nonendog.	Unclassifiable
< 1500	6	4	10	5	1	3
> 1500	3	0	2	11	12	6

Chi square including all groups = 22.64, p < 0.001.
Chi square excluding unclassifiable group = 21.85, p < 0.001.

TABLE III
Norepinephrine (NE) and normetanephrine (NMN) excretion in subtypes of depressive disorders

Depressive Subtype	NE (μg/24 hrs)	NMN (μg/24 hrs)
Schizophrenia-Related	33 ± 7	214 ± 44
Schizoaffective	23 ± 4	285 ± 34
Bipolar Manic-Depressive	27 ± 4	225 ± 26
Unipolar Endogenous	45 ± 4	323 ± 43
Unipolar Nonendogenous	39 ± 6	247 ± 27
Unclassifiable	41 ± 4	209 ± 12

Urinary catecholamines and metabolites were determined in two to ten separate 24-hour urine samples obtained from each patient. The average value for each patient was used to compute the group means and standard errors of the means presented in this table.

schizophrenia-related depressions, in the schizoaffective depressions, and in the bipolar manic-depressive depressions.

Although MHPG was the only catecholamine metabolite that showed a pronounced and statistically significant difference in levels when values in bipolar manic-depressive and unipolar nonendogenous depressions were compared, we could not rule out the possibility that the other urinary metabolites might also contain information which would be useful in differentiating these two types of depressive disorders. In order to explore this possibility further, multivariate discriminant function analysis (15) was applied to the biochemical data obtained from an initial series of patients with bipolar manic-depressive and unipolar nonendogenous depressions.

The terms available to the computer for entry into the discrimination equation included: norepinephrine, normetanephrine, epinephrine, metanephrine, VMA, MHPG, and various sums and ratios of these terms. Using these terms, a discrimination equation was developed in a stepwise procedure, where the variable selected by the computer for entry into the equation at each step was the one

Biochemical Subgroups

TABLE IV
Epinephrine (E) and metanephrine (MN) excretion
in subtypes of depressive disorders

Depressive Subtype	E (μg/24 hrs)	MN (μg/24 hrs)
Schizophrenia-Related	5.5 ± 1.0*	72 ± 14**
Schizoaffective	10.2 ± 0.8	224 ± 15
Bipolar Manic-Depressive	8.2 ± 1.2	161 ± 19
Unipolar Endogenous	9.8 ± 1.0	144 ± 11
Unipolar Nonendogenous	10.3 ± 1.4	168 ± 16
Unclassifiable	9.5 ± 1.6	137 ± 74

See caption to Table III.
* $p < 0.05$;
** $p < 0.01$ compared to unipolar nonendogenous group.

with the largest contribution to discrimination. As shown in Table VI, the equation was of the form: Depression Type (D-Type) score =

$$C_1 (MHPG) + C_2 (VMA) + C_3 (NE) + C_4 \frac{(NMN + MN)}{(VMA)} + C_0$$

In developing the metric for this equation a value of 0 was assigned to bipolar manic-depressive depressions, and a value of 1 was assigned to unipolar nonendogenous depressions. Therefore, in the application of this equation, D-type scores less than 0.5 were associated with bipolar manic-depressive depressions and D-type scores greater than 0.5 were associated with unipolar nonendogenous depressions.

This equation was then applied to data on urinary catecholamines and metabolites obtained from an independent series of depressed patients who were studied after the derivation of this equation, and whose biochemical data, therefore, had not been used to derive the parameters of the equation.

Psychotropic Drug Research

TABLE V
VMA and MHPG excretion
in subtypes of depressive disorders

Depressive Subtype	VMA (μg/24 hrs)	MHPG (μg/24 hrs)
Schizophrenia-Related	3633 ± 385	1403 ± 141*
Schizoaffective	3806 ± 279	1149 ± 125**
Bipolar Manic-Depressive	4041 ± 211	1209 ± 89***
Unipolar Endogenous	3782 ± 246	1950 ± 177
Unipolar Nonendogenous	3540 ± 232	1814 ± 92
Unclassifiable	3863 ± 207	1815 ± 171

See caption to Table III.
* $p < 0.05$;
** $p < 0.01$;
*** $p < 0.001$ compared to unipolar nonendogenous group.

As shown in Figure 2 and Table VII, all of the patients with independent clinical diagnoses of bipolar manic-depressive or schizoaffective depressions in the validation sample had D-type scores below 0.5. In contrast, all of the patients with diagnoses of unipolar nonendogenous depressions as well as all patients with schizophrenia-related depressions and unclassifiable depressions had D-type scores greater than 0.5. While most of the patients with unipolar endogenous depressions had D-type scores greater than 0.5, several of these patients had D-type scores below 0.5, that is, in the range observed in the bipolar manic-depressive or schizoaffective depressions. Thus, D-type scores below 0.5 may conceivably help to identify, from within the overall group of unipolar endogenous depressions, those patients with a biochemical similarity or predisposition to bipolar manic-depressive (or schizoaffective) disorders, even though the patient may not have had a history of prior overt episodes of hypomania or mania or other forms of excited states.

In order to evaluate the contribution of each of the terms in the

Biochemical Subgroups

TABLE VI

Discrimination equation for D-type score

Coefficients and Constant	Standardized Coefficients
$C_1 = 3.734 \times 10^{-4}$	0.438
$C_2 = -2.303 \times 10^{-4}$	-0.454
$C_3 = 1.035 \times 10^{-2}$	0.420
$C_4 = -4.217$	-0.389
$C_0 = 0.918$	———

All of the biochemical variables that appear in this equation are expressed in $\mu g/24$ hrs. The standardized coefficients which apply to normalized data (mean = 0, standard deviation = 1) show the relative contributions of each term without metric differences.

D-Type Score =

$$C_1 (\text{MHPG}) + C_2 (\text{VMA}) + C_3 (\text{NE}) + C_4 \frac{(\text{NMN} + \text{MN})}{(\text{VMA})} + C_0$$

four-term discrimination equation, we derive discrimination equations based on one, two, and three as well as all four of the terms, using the biochemical data obtained from the initial series of patients with bipolar manic-depressive and unipolar nonendogenous depressions. D-type scores based on these equations were then generated for depressed patients in the validation sample whose biochemical data had not been used to derive the equations.

As shown in Figure 3, the one-term equation (based on MHPG alone) tended to separate these groups but there was some overlap. The two-term equation (based on MHPG and VMA) provided better discrimination between the groups, but some overlap remained. The three-term equation (based on MHPG, VMA, and norepinephrine) removed all overlap between the two groups but a fair number of subjects were still clustered around the centroid of 0.5. The four-term equation (based on MHPG, VMA, NE, and the ratio $\frac{(\text{NMN} + \text{MN})}{(\text{VMA})}$ improved upon the discrimination by providing a very wide separation of the D-type scores in these two groups without any overlap. It should be re-emphasized that these groups were comprised only of patients from the validation sample whose biochemical data had not been used to derive these equations.

9

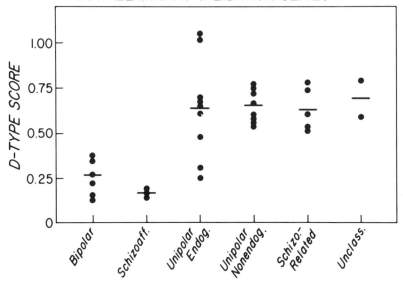

D-TYPE SCORES (FOUR TERM)
FOR ALL DEPRESSED PATIENTS
IN PRELIMINARY VALIDATION SERIES

FIGURE 2   D-type scores (four term) for all depressed patients in preliminary validation series. D-type scores were computed using the biochemical data from two to six separate 24-hour urine samples obtained from
each patient. The mean D-type score for each patient was plotted. The
overall mean for each subgroup is indicated by a horizontal line (—) drawn
through the data points.

Although additional studies, using a larger sample of patients, are
needed to further validate and refine the four-term discrimination
equation for obtaining D-type scores, the present findings suggest
that this equation may provide an even more precise discrimination
among biologically meaningful subtypes of depressive disorders
than does urinary MHPG alone. Thus, it is intriguing to speculate
that the discrimination equation, by including the contribution of
various urinary catecholamine metabolites of peripheral origin, may
be correcting for that fraction of urinary MHPG that derives from
the periphery rather than from the brain.

Table VIII presents data from patients on whom four-term D-
type scores and measures of platelet MAO activity were obtained
concurrently. As shown in Table VIII, platelet MAO activity was

TABLE VII

Distribution of D-type scores for all depressed patients
in preliminary validation series

D-Type Score	Bipolar Manic-Dep.	Schizo-affective	Unipolar Endog.	Unipolar Nonendog.	Schizo-Related	Unclassifiable
< 0.5	6	3	3	0	0	0
> 0.5	0	0	6	8	5	2

Chi square = 24.36; $p < 0.001$.

Psychotropic Drug Research

D-TYPE SCORES COMPUTED USING ONE, TWO, THREE AND FOUR TERM DISCRIMINATION EQUATIONS : PRELIMINARY VALIDATION SERIES

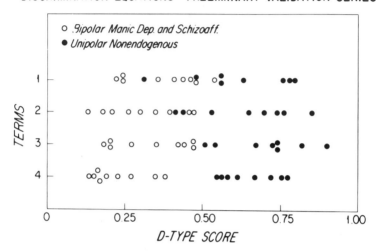

FIGURE 3   D-type scores computed using one, two, three, and four term discrimination equations: preliminary validation series. The following equations were generated from the body of data that was initially used to derive the original four-term (D-type) discrimination equation:

D-type score (1 term) = 3.916×10^{-4} (MHPG) $- 0.104$

D-type score (2 term) = 4.352×10^{-4} (MHPG) $- 0.996 \times 10^{-4}$ (VMA) $+ 0.913$

D-type score (3 term) = 3.606×10^{-4} (MHPG) $- 1.297 \times 10^{-4}$ (VMA) $+ 0.671 \times 10^{-2}$ (NE) $+ 0.203$

D-type score (4 term) = 3.734×10^{-4} (MHPG) $- 2.303 \times 10^{-4}$ (VMA) $+ 1.035 \times 10^{-2}$ (NE) $- 4.217 \dfrac{\text{(NMN + MN)}}{\text{(VMA)}} + 0.918$

significantly lower in depressed patients with D-type scores less than 0.5 than in depressed patients with D-type scores greater than 0.5. These findings showing that patients with low versus high D-type scores have a significant difference in an independent bio-chemical measure further suggest that the D-type score may be dis-criminating among biologically meaningful subgroups of depressive disorders. Moreover, the data in this slide are consistent with pre-vious findings of other investigators (33, 24, 25), who have found reductions in platelet MAO activity in patients with bipolar manic-depressive disorders, i.e., a depressive subtype that we have found to have low D-type scores.

12

Biochemical Subgroups

TABLE VIII
Platelet MAO activity in depressed patients
with D-type scores below and above 0.5

D-Type Score	N	Platelet MAO Activity
< 0.5	5	3.28 ± 0.60*
> 0.5	9	6.73 ± 0.56*

Platelet MAO activity was determined in up to 3 separate blood samples obtained from each patient. The average value for each patient was used to compute the group means and standard errors of the means presented in this Table. Platelet MAO activity is expressed in nanomoles of tryptamine deaminated/hr/mg platelet protein.
N = number of patients.
* p < 0.005 for difference between groups.

In another aspect of our research, we too have been examining platelet MAO activity in patients with psychiatric disorders. Table IX summarizes aspects of our data on platelet MAO activity in patients with unipolar endogenous and schizophrenia-related depressions (i.e., depressive disorders characterized clinically by the presence of chronic asocial, eccentric, or bizarre behavior). The findings in Table IX show that patients with schizophrenia-related depressions had significantly higher platelet MAO activity than did control subjects or patients with unipolar endogenous depressions. Our findings of an increase in platelet MAO activity in patients with schizophrenia-related depressions appear consistent with the observations of Brockington and associates (9) who reported an increase in platelet MAO activity in those patients who concurrently met those investigators' criteria for both schizophrenic and affective disorders. Moreover, in considering our findings of elevated platelet MAO activity in the schizophrenia-related depres-

TABLE IX
Platelet MAO activity in unipolar endogenous
and schizophrenia-related depressions

Group	N	Age	MAO Activity
Controls	28	27 ± 1	5.72 ± 0.38
Uni. Endog. Dep.	13	42 ± 4	5.87 ± 0.64
Schiz.-Rel. Dep.	8	27 ± 4	8.16 ± 0.53*

* p < 0.025 for difference from the control or unipolar endogenous groups.

sions (characterized by chronic asocial behavior), it is of some interest to note that Redmond and Murphy (39), in studies of platelet MAO activity in the rhesus monkey, found that platelet MAO activity showed statistically significant positive correlations with time spent alone, inactivity, and passivity, and statistically significant negative (inverse) correlations with social contact, ambulatory movement, and (in males only) play. Thus, it may be that social isolation is the variable that correlates with elevated platelet MAO activity.

In summary, as shown in Table X, the findings presented in this section of the paper suggest that we can discriminate three biochemically discrete subgroups of depressive disorders. Subgroup I, which is characterized biochemically by low urinary MHPG excretion, low D-type scores, and low urinary norepinephrine (as well as low platelet MAO activity) includes the clinically defined subtypes that we diagnose as bipolar manic-depressive depressions and schizoaffective depressions as well as some of the so-called uni-

TABLE X

Summary of three biochemically discrete subgroups of depressive disorders tentatively identified in our studies

Subgroup	Biochemical Characteristics	Clinical Subtypes of Depressions Included
I.	Low Urinary MHPG Low D-type Scores (< 0.5) Low Urinary Norepinephrine	Bipolar Manic-Depressive Schizoaffective Some Unipolar Endogenous
II.	High Urinary MHPG High D-type Scores (> 0.5)	Unipolar Nonendogenous Some Unipolar Endogenous
III.	Low Urinary MHPG High D-type Scores (> 0.5) Low Urinary Epinephrine Low Urinary Metanephrine High Platelet MAO Activity	Schizophrenia- Related

polar endogenous depressions.

In contrast, subgroup II is characterized biochemically by high urinary MHPG excretion and high D-type scores and includes the unipolar nonendogenous depressions and most of the patients we diagnose as unipolar endogenous depressions (Table X).

As shown in Table X, subgroup III is characterized biochemically by low urinary MHPG, high D-type scores, low urinary epinephrine, low urinary metanephrine, and high platelet MAO activity. This subgroup includes patients whom we diagnose clinically as schizophrenia-related depressions.

Thus, our data suggest that we now can discriminate biochemically discrete subgroups of depressive disorders on the basis of measurements of urinary catecholamines and metabolites as well as platelet MAO activity. Further research is currently in progress to confirm and extend these findings.

III. BIOCHEMICAL DISCRIMINATION OF SUBGROUPS OF SCHIZOPHRENIC AND SCHIZOPHRENIA-RELATED DISORDERS

Since the initial report of Murphy and Wyatt (34), a number of studies have now confirmed that some patients with schizophrenic disorders have lower platelet monoamine oxidase activity than controls (63,32,36,65,13,46,5,56); but this has not been observed in other studies (16,54,57,9,4,59). It has been noted that reduced platelet monoamine oxidase activity occurs more commonly in chronic than in acute schizophrenic disorders (11). However, since other clinical characteristics that may be associated with reduced platelet MAO activity in schizophrenic patients had not been demonstrated, and because of our interest in possible biochemical discriminators of subtypes of schizophrenic and affective disorders (including the schizophrenia-related depressions), several years ago we initiated a series of studies to explore this problem.*

In a pilot study of platelet MAO activity in schizophrenic patients hospitalized at the Massachusetts Mental Health Center or the McLean Hospital, we first noted that reduced platelet MAO activity regularly occurred in a subgroup of schizophrenic patients (most of whom were paranoid) with auditory hallucinations and delusions. In order to confirm this initial observation, we examined platelet MAO activity in a subsequent series of patients hospi-

*Preliminary findings from these studies were presented in 1975 at the Annual Meeting of The American Psychiatric Association, Anaheim, California (45), and have been reported in brief communications elsewhere (46,51).

talized at the Massachusetts Mental Health Center with a diagnosis of schizophrenia made in accordance with the American Psychiatric Association, Diagnostic and Statistical Manual of Mental Disorders (1). In this aspect of our research we excluded patients with prominent affective symptoms of depressions or manias. As shown in Table XI, mean platelet MAO activity was lower in the group of 32 nonaffective schizophrenic patients (i.e., schizophrenic patients without prominent affective symptoms of depressions or manias) than in an age-matched control group (p < .05).

TABLE XI
Platelet MAO activity in schizophrenics
and controls

Group	N	Age	MAO Activity
Controls	28	27 ± 1	5.72 ± 0.38
Schizophrenics	32	27 ± 1	4.70 ± 0.31*

Platelet MAO activity is expressed as means ± S.E.M. in nanomoles of tryptamine deaminated/hr/mg protein. Age is expressed as means ± S.E.M. in years.
* p < 0.05 for difference from control values.

The medical records of these schizophrenic patients were then reviewed in detail by a psychiatrist blind to the biochemical data, and the patients were categorized according to whether they had a well documented record of both auditory hallucinations and delusions. The subgroup of schizophrenic patients with both documented auditory hallucinations and delusions was designated S-2, whereas the remaining subgroup of schizophrenic patients was designated S-1. Most of the male patients and half of the female patients in the S-2 subgroup had delusions or auditory hallucinations that were of a persecutory or accusatory nature, and thus were also classified as paranoid.

As shown in Table XII, patients with a diagnosis of schizophrenia but without documented auditory hallucinations and delusions (the S-1 subgroup) had platelet MAO activity that was very similar to that of the control group. In contrast, schizophrenic patients with both auditory hallucinations and delusions (the S-2 subgroup) had significantly (p < 0.001) lower platelet MAO activity (Table XII). There was relatively little overlap of individual values of platelet MAO activity in patients in the two schizophrenic subgroups. Within the S-2 subgroup, the lowest individual values of platelet MAO activity were observed in patients who were paranoid, as suggested

Biochemical Subgroups

TABLE XII
Platelet MAO activity in schizophrenic
subgroups and controls

Group	N	Age	MAO Activity
Controls	28	27 ± 1	5.72 ± 0.38
S-1	16	26 ± 1	5.95 ± 0.35
S-2	16	29 ± 2	3.45 ± 0.27*

See caption to Table XI.
* $p < 0.001$ for difference from controls or S-1 subgroup.

by observations made in our earlier pilot study.

The S-1 and S-2 subgroups did not differ significantly in age or sex distribution. However, to rule out the possibility that sex differences might be contributing to these differences in platelet MAO activity, the data on male and female patients were examined separately. As shown in Table XIII, both the male and female schizophrenic subgroups were well matched to controls for age; although the S-2 subgroup did tend to be a few years older than the S-1 subgroup, the difference was not significant. In both male and female patients, platelet MAO activity was significantly lower in the S-2 subgroup than in the S-1 subgroup or the controls (Table XIII).

Since it had been suggested that reduced platelet MAO activity may occur principally in chronic schizophrenic patients, we examined several measures that might reflect chronicity. In this series of schizophrenic patients, platelet MAO activity was not related to

TABLE XIII
Platelet MAO activity in schizophrenic subgroups:
male and female patients

Sex	Subgroup	N	Age	MAO Activity
Male	Control	14	28 ± 2	5.78 ± 0.67
	S-1	8	26 ± 1	6.06 ± 0.49
	S-2	8	30 ± 3	2.86 ± 0.30**
Female	Control	14	26 ± 1	5.66 ± 0.41
	S-1	8	26 ± 3	5.86 ± 0.53
	S-2	8	27 ± 2	4.04 ± 0.35*

See caption to Table XI.
* $p < 0.02$;
** $p < 0.01$ for difference from respective controls or S-1 subgroups.

the number of previous hospitalizations or to the length of time since the first documented hospital admission, thus suggesting that reduced platelet MAO activity in the S-2 subgroup was not merely related to chronicity of the illness. Since it was not feasible to conduct this aspect of our research on schizophrenic patients under drug-free conditions, the comparison between the S-1 and S-2 subgroups provides some control for possible effects of antipsychotic drugs, since many of the patients in both groups were treated with these drugs. Moreover, in this series of patients, MAO activity was not meaningfully correlated with antipsychotic drug dosage ($r = -.09$). Similarly, Wyatt and Murphy (62) have not observed changes in platelet MAO activity resulting from administration of phenothiazine antipsychotic agents.

While (in this study) we excluded those schizophrenic patients with prominent affective symptomatology, in another aspect of this work, as described above (Section I—Biochemical Discrimination of Subgroups of Affective Disorders), we have also examined platelet MAO activity in a series of depressed patients with diagnoses of schizophrenia-related depressions, characterized by the presence of chronic asocial, eccentric, or bizarre behavior.* These patients were studied during a period of clinical depression at a time when they were receiving no psychoactive drugs. As was noted above (see Table IX), patients with schizophrenia-related depressions had significantly higher platelet MAO activity than did a group of age-matched control subjects, or a group of patients with unipolar endogenous depressions who were somewhat older. It is interesting to note that patients with schizophrenia-related depressions did not differ significantly from patients with nonaffective schizophrenic disorders (i.e., the S-1 and S-2 subgroups) in the number of hospitalizations, the time since first hospital admission, and the age at first hospital admission. Platelet MAO activity in the patients with unipolar endogenous depressions did not differ from control values (see Table IX). Since most of the patients with schizophrenia-related depressions were female, the data on female patients and control subjects were examined separately, and the findings were similar.

The findings of this study indicate that reduced platelet MAO activity is not found in all schizophrenic patients, but that it tends to occur in a clinically identifiable subgroup. The original blind selection of the S-2 subgroup was made on the basis of a history of

*Patients with schizoaffective depressions characterized by affect nonconsonant delusions or hallucinations occurring in the absence of a history of chronic asocial, eccentric, or bizarre behavior were not included in this diagnostic group.

both auditory hallucinations and delusions. However, further examination of our data suggested that the primary discriminating symptom may have been the presence of auditory hallucinations, since none of the patients in the S-1 subgroup had auditory hallucinations although many had delusions. Thus, it is possible that our S-2 subgroup may correspond to the schizophrenic subtypes identified in other studies on the basis of auditory hallucinations (61).

Our findings thus suggest that, in schizophrenic patients without prominent affective symptomatology, the presence of auditory hallucinations, particularly in conjunction with paranoid features, may be a sufficient criterion for identifying a subgroup of schizophrenic disorders with reduced platelet MAO activity. Although further prospective studies will be required to confirm this, recent data from several other laboratories have provided some preliminary confirmation of our results. Following the initial report (45) and publication of our findings (46), two groups of investigators reanalyzed their own data on platelet MAO activity in schizophrenic patients, and found lower platelet MAO activity in patients with auditory hallucinations than in patients without such hallucinations (3, and Meltzer—personal communication). Moreover, in their series of schizophrenic patients, Wyatt and his colleagues have found that patients with paranoid schizophrenic disorders had lower platelet MAO activity than did nonparanoid schizophrenic patients (64).

In summary, as shown in Figure 4, we have observed the following: a) mean platelet MAO activity is not different from control values in the subgroup of nonaffective schizophrenic disorders without auditory hallucinations (S-1 subgroup), b) mean platelet MAO activity is reduced in the subgroup of nonaffective schizophrenic disorders characterized by the presence of auditory hallucinations in conjunction with paranoid features (S-2 subgroup), and c) mean platelet MAO activity is increased in schizophrenia-related depressions. Thus, our data suggest that the schizophrenia-related depressive disorders may be distinguished biochemically from subgroups of nonaffective schizophrenic disorders as well as from other subgroups of depressive disorders.

These findings of differences in platelet MAO activity in these clinically defined subgroups of nonaffective schizophrenic disorders and the schizophrenia-related depressive disorders may help to account for some of the discrepancies in findings among the various studies of platelet MAO activity in schizophrenic and affective

19

Psychotropic Drug Research

PLATELET MAO ACTIVITY IN SCHIZOPHRENIC SUBGROUPS AND SCHIZOPHRENIA-RELATED DEPRESSIONS

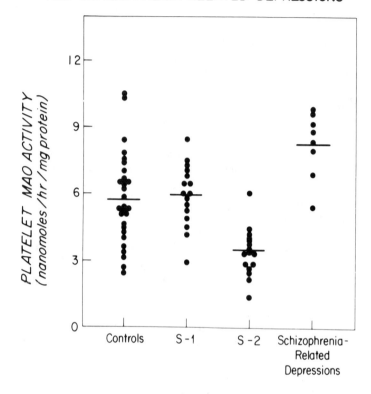

FIGURE 4   Platelet MAO activity in subgroups of nonaffective schizophrenic disorders and in schizophrenia-related depressions. This figure summarizes the major findings on platelet MAO activity reported in the text. Each point represents the data from one patient or control subject. The mean value for each subgroup is indicated by a horizontal line (—) drawn through the data points.

disorders, as reviewed above. Further studies in a larger series of patients are now in progress to confirm and extend these findings.

IV. CONCLUDING SUMMARY

The urinary excretion of MHPG and other catecholamine metabolites was measured in a series of patients with various clinically defined subtypes of depressive disorders. MHPG excretion was significantly lower in bipolar manic-depressive depressions and in

20

schizoaffective depressions than in unipolar nonendogenous depressions. Patients with schizophrenia-related depressions also excreted reduced levels of MHPG when compared with unipolar nonendogenous depressions. Levels of urinary epinephrine and metanephrine also were significantly reduced in patients with schizophrenia-related depressions, and these patients, moreover, had higher levels of platelet MAO activity than control subjects or patients with unipolar endogenous depressions.

In these studies we also found that further biochemical discrimination among depressive subtypes is provided by the following equation, derived empirically by applying multivariate discriminant function analysis to data on urinary catecholamine metabolites: Depression-type (D-type) score =

$$C_1\,(\text{MHPG}) + C_2\,(\text{VMA}) + C_3\,(\text{NE}) + C_4\,\frac{(\text{NMN} + \text{MN})}{(\text{VMA})} + C_0$$

In the original derivation of this equation, low scores were related to bipolar manic-depressive depressions, and high scores were related to unipolar nonendogenous (chronic characterological) depressions. Findings from a series of depressed patients whose biochemical data had not been used to derive this equation confirmed these differences in D-type scores among subtypes of depressions. The data presented in this paper suggest that we can discriminate three biochemically discrete subgroups of depressive disorders.

In another aspect of our research, platelet monoamine oxidase (MAO) activity was measured in patients with nonaffective schizophrenic disorders (i.e., without prominent symptoms of depressions or manias) and in patients with schizophrenia-related depressions. MAO activity was significantly lower than control values in a subgroup of patients with nonaffective schizophrenic disorders (most of whom were paranoid) characterized by the presence of auditory hallucinations and delusions. Platelet MAO activity was not reduced in the subgroup of nonaffective schizophrenic patients without auditory hallucinations. These findings of differences in platelet MAO activity in clinically defined subgroups of nonaffective schizophrenic disorders as well as in the schizophrenia-related depressive disorders may help to account for some of the discrepancies in findings among the various studies of platelet MAO activity in schizophrenic and affective disorders.

In summary, these studies, showing differences in a number of biochemical measures in different clinically defined subtypes of

Psychotropic Drug Research

affective and schizophrenic disorders, suggest that these biochemical measurements may help to distinguish clinically relevant, biologically discrete subgroups of psychiatric disorders. While additional confirmation and extension of these findings is required, this work may well represent the initial steps in the development of a psychiatric nosology that is based not only upon descriptive clinical phenomenology, but also upon a knowledge of the biochemical pathophysiology underlying these phenomena. Exploration of the therapeutic implications and pharmacological relevance of such a biochemical classification of psychiatric disorders presents both a major challenge, and what could prove to be one of the most productive and clinically beneficial areas for future research in the entire field of psychopharmacology.

ACKNOWLEDGMENTS

The authors wish to thank Mr. Edwin Grab, Ms. Patricia Platz Kizuka, Mrs. Sandra Lipchus, Mrs. Mary McLellan and Ms. Ellen Kruger for their technical assistance in the conduct of this research.

REFERENCES

1. American Psychiatric Association. *Diagnostic and Statistical Manual of Mental Disorders*, 2nd edition, Washington, D.C., 1968.
2. Axelrod, J., Kopin, I.J. and Mann, J.D.: 3-Methoxy-4-hydroxyphenylglycol sulfate, a new metabolite of epinephrine and norepinephrine. *Biochem. Biophys. Acta* 36:576-577, 1959.
3. Becker, R.E. and Shaskan, E.G.: Platelet monoamine oxidase activity in schizophrenic patients. *Am. J. Psychiat.* 134:512-517, 1977.
4. Belmaker, R.H., Ebbesen, K., Ebstein, R. and Rimon, R.: Platelet monoamine oxidase in schizophrenia and manic-depressive illness. *Br. J. Psychiat.* 129:227-232, 1976.
5. Berrettini, W.H., Vogel, W.H., and Clouse, R.: Monoamine oxidase in chronic schizophrenia. *Am. J. Psychiat.* 134:805-806, 1977.
6. Bond, P.A., Dimitrakoudi, M., Howlett, D.R. and Jenner, F.A.: Urinary excretion of the sulfate and glucuronide of 3-methoxy-4-hydroxyphenylethyleneglycol in a manic-depressive patient. *Psychol. Med.* 5: 279-285, 1975.
7. Bond, P.A., Jenner, F.A. and Sampson, G.A.: Daily variations of the urine content of 3-methoxy-4-hydroxyphenylglycol in two manic-depressive patients. *Psychol. Med.* 2:81-85, 1972.
8. Breese, G.R., Prange, A.J., Jr., Howard, J.L., Lipton, M.A., McKinney, W.T., Bowman, R.E. and Bushnell, P.: 3-Methoxy-4-hydroxyphenylglycol excretion and behavioral changes in rat and monkey after central sympathectomy with 6-hydroxydopamine. *Nature New*

Biol. 240:286-287, 1972.

9. Brockington, I., Crow, T.J., Johnstone, E.C. and Owens, F.: An investigation of platelet monoamine oxidase activity in schizophrenia and schizoaffective psychosis, In G.E.W. Wolston-holme and J. Knight (Eds.), *Monoamine Oxidase and Its Inhibitors,* CIBA Symp. #39 (New Series), Elsevier, New York, 1976, pp. 353-369.

10. Bunney, W.E., Jr., Goodwin, F.K., Murphy, D.L., House, K.M. and Gordon, E.K.: The "switch process" in manic-depressive illness. *Arch. Gen. Psychiatry* 27:304-309, 1972.

11. Carpenter, W.T., Murphy, D.L. and Wyatt, R.J.: Platelet monoamine oxidase activity in acute schizophrenia. *Am. J. Psychiat.* 132: 438-441, 1975.

12. DeLeon-Jones, F.D., Maas, J.W., Dekirmenjian, H. and Fawcett, J.A.: Urinary catecholamine metabolites during behavioral changes in a patient with manic-depressive cycles. *Science* 179:300-302, 1973.

13. Domino, E.F. and Khanna, S.S.: Decreased blood platelet MAO activity in unmedicated chronic schizophrenic patients. *Am. J. Psychiat.* 133:323-326, 1976.

14. Ebert, M.H. and Kopin, I.J.: Differential labelling of origins of urinary catecholamine metabolites by dopamine-C[14]. *Trans. Assoc. Am. Physicians* 28:256-264, 1975.

15. Fisher, R.A.: The use of multiple measurements in taxonomic problems. *Ann. Eugenics* 7:179-188, 1936.

16. Friedman, E., Shopsin, B., Sathananthan, G. and Gershon, S.: Blood platelet monoamine oxidase activity in psychiatric patients. *Am. J. Psychiatry* 131:1392-1394, 1974.

17. Garfinkel, P.E., Warsh, J.J., Stancer, H.C. and Godse, D.D.: Urinary 3-methoxy-4-hydroxyphenylglycol in bipolar illness after carbidopa. *American Psychiatric Association New Research Abstracts,* 1976, p. 7.

18. Glowinski, J., Kopin, I.J. and Axelrod, J.: Metabolism of H[3]-norepinephrine in rat brain. *J. Neurochem.* 12:25-30, 1965.

19. Goodwin, F.K. and Post, R.M.: Studies of amine metabolites in affective illness and in schizophrenia: a comparative analysis, In D.X. Freedman, (Ed.), *Biology of the Major Psychoses,* Raven Press, New York, 1975, pp. 299-332.

20. Greenspan, K., Schildkraut, J.J., Gordon, E.K., Levy, B. and Durell, J.: Catecholamine metabolism in affective disorders III. MHPG and other catecholamine metabolites in patients treated with lithium carbonate. *J. Psychiatry Res.* 7:171-183, 1970.

21. Hamilton M: A rating scale for depression. *J. Neurol. Neurosurg. Psychiatry* 23:56-62, 1960.

22. Hoeldtke, R.D., Rogawski, M. and Wurtman, R.J.: Effects of selective destruction of central and peripheral catecholamine containing neurons with 6-hydroxydopamine on catecholamine excretion in the rat. *Br. J. Pharmacol.* 50:265-270, 1974.

23. Karoum, F., Wyatt, R. and Costa, E.: Estimation of the contribution of peripheral and central noradrenaline neurons to urinary 3-methoxy-4-hydroxyphenylglycol in the rat. *Neuropharmacology* 13:165-176, 1974.
24. Landowski, J., Lysiak, W. and Angielski, S.: Monoamine oxidase activity in blood platelets from patients with cyclophrenic depressive syndromes. *Biochem. Med.* 14:347-354, 1975.
25. Leckman, J.F., Gershon, E.S., Nichols, A.S. and Murphy, D.L.: Reduced MAO activity in first-degree relatives of individuals with bipolar affective disorders. *Arch. Gen. Psychiatry* 34:601-606, 1977.
26. Maas, J.W. and Hattox, S.E.: Determination of neurotransmitter metabolite production by brain in awake man. Presented at the Fourth International Catecholamine Symposium — *Catecholamines: Basic and Clinical Frontiers*, Asilomar, California, September, 1978.
27. Maas, J.W. and Landis, D.H.: *In vivo* studies of metabolism of norepinephrine in central nervous system. *J. Pharmacol. Exper. Ther.* 163:147-162, 1968.
28. Maas, J. W., Dekirmenjian, H. and DeLeon-Jones, F.: The identification of depressed patients who have a disorder of norepinephrine metabolism and/or disposition, In E. Usdin, and S. Snyder, (Eds.), *Frontiers in Catecholamine Research*, Pergamon Press, New York, 1973, pp. 1091-1096.
29. Maas, J.W., Dekirmenjian, H., Garver, D., Redmond, D.E., Jr., and Landis, D.H.: Catecholamine metabolite excretion following intraventricular injection of 6-OH-dopamine. *Brain Res.* 41: 507-511, 1972.
30. Maas, J.W., Fawcett, J.A. and Dekirmenjian, H.: Catecholamine metabolism, depressive illness and drug response. *Arch. Gen. Psychiatry* 26:252-262, 1972.
31. Mannarino, E., Kirshner, N. and Nashold, B. S., Jr.: Metabolism of C^{14}-noradrenaline by cat brain *in vivo. J. Neurochem.* 12:25-30, 1965.
32. Meltzer, H.Y. and Stahl, S. M.: Platelet monoamine oxidase activity and substrate preferences in schizophrenic patients. *Res. Comm. Chem. Path. Pharmacol.* 7:419-431, 1974.
33. Murphy, D. L. and Weiss, R.: Reduced monoamine oxidase activity in blood platelet from bipolar depressed patients. *Am. J. Psychiatry* 128:1351-1357, 1972.
34. Murphy, D.L. and Wyatt, R. J.: Reduced monoamine oxidase activity in blood platelets from schizophrenic patients. *Nature* 238:225-226, 1972.
35. Muscettola, G., Wehr, T. and Goodwin, F. K.: Central norepinephrine responses in depression versus normals. *American Psychiatric Association New Research Abstracts*, p. 8, 1976.
36. Nies, A., Robinson, D.S., Harris, L.S. and Lamborn, K.R.: Comparison of monoamine oxidase substrate activities in twins, schizophrenics, depressives and controls, In E. Usdin (Ed.), *Neuropsychopharmacology of Monoamines and Their Regulatory Enzymes*, Raven Press,

New York, 1974, pp. 59-70.
37. Orsulak, P.J., Schildkraut, J.J., Schatzberg, A. F. and Herzog, J. M.: Differences in platelet monoamine oxidase activity in subgroups of schizophrenic and depressive disorders. *Biol. Psychiatry* 13:637-647, 1978.
38. Post, R.M., Stoddard, F.J., Gillin, J.C., Buchsbaum, M.D., Runkle, D.C., Black, K.E. and Bunney, W.E., Jr.: Alterations in motor activity, sleep, and biochemistry in a cycling manic-depressive patient. *Arch. Gen. Psychiatry* 34:470-477, 1977.
39. Redmond, D.E., Jr. and Murphy, D.L.: Behavioral correlates of platelet monoamine oxidase activity in rhesus monkeys. *Psychosom. Med.* 37:80, 1976.
40. Rutledge, C.O. and Jonason, J.: Metabolic pathways of dopamine and norepinephrine in rabbit brain *in vitro. J. Pharmcol. Exper. Ther.* 157:493-502, 1967.
41. Schanberg, S.M., Breese, G.R., Schildkraut, J.J., Gordon, E.K. and Kopin, I.J.: 3-Methoxy-4-hydroxyphenylglycol sulfate in brain and cerebrospinal fluid. *Biochem. Pharmacol.* 17:2006-2008, 1968.
42. Schanberg, S.M., Schildkraut, J.J., Breese, G.R. and Kopin, I.J.: Metabolism of normetanephrine-H[3] in rat brain—identification of conjugated 3-methoxy-4-hydroxyphenylglycol as major metabolite. *Biochem. Pharmacol.* 17:247-254, 1968.
43. Schildkraut, J.J.: The catecholamine hypothesis of affective disorders: a review of supporting evidence. *Am. J. Psychiatry* 122:509-522, 1965.
44. Schildkraut, J.J.: Catecholamine metabolism and affective disorders: studies of MHPG excretion, In E. Usdin, and S. Snyder (Eds.), *Frontiers in Catecholamine Research,* Pergamon Press, New York, 1973, pp. 1165-1171.
45. Schildkraut, J.J., Herzog, J.M., Edelman, S.E., Frazier, S.H., Shein, H.M. and Orsulak, P.J.: Platelet MAO Activity in Schizophrenic Disorders. *American Psychiatric Association New Research Abstracts,* Annual Meeting, Anaheim, California, 1975, p. 22.
46. Schildkraut, J.J., Herzog, J.M., Orsulak, P.J., Edelman, S.E., Shein, H.M. and Frazier, S.H.: Reduced platelet monoamine oxidase activity in a subgroup of schizophrenic patients. *Am. J. Psychiatry* 133:438-440, 1976.
47. Schildkraut, J.J., Keeler, B.A., Grab, E.L., Kantrowich, J. and Hartmann, E.: MHPG excretion and clinical classification in depressive disorders. *Lancet I*:1251-1252, 1973.
48. Schildkraut, J.J., Keeler, B.A., Papousek, M. and Hartmann, E.: MHPG excretion in depressive disorders: relation to clinical subtypes and desynchronized sleep. *Science* 181:762-764, 1973.
49. Schildkraut, J.J., Keeler, B.A., Rogers, M.P. and Draskoczy, P.R.: Catecholamine metabolism in affective disorders: a longitudinal study of a patient treated with amitriptyline and ECT. *Psychosomatic Medicine* 34:470 (Abstract); plus erratum *Psychosomatic Medicine*

35:274, 1973.

50. Schildkraut, J.J., Orsulak, P.J., LaBrie, R.A., Schatzberg, A.F., Gudeman, J.E., Cole, J.O. and Rohde, W.A.: Towards a biochemical classification of depressive disorders II: application of multivariate discriminant function analysis to data on urinary catecholamines and metabolites. *Arch. Gen. Psychiatry*, 35:1436-1439, 1978.

51. Schildkraut, J.J., Orsulak, P.J., Schatzberg, A.F., Cole, J.O., Gudeman, J.E. and Rohde, W.A.: Elevated platelet monoamine oxidase (MAO) activity in schizophrenia-related depressive disorders. *Am.J. Psychiatry.* 135:110-112, 1978.

52. Schildkraut, J.J., Orsulak, P.J., Schatzberg, A.F., Gudeman, J.E., Cole, J.O., Rohde, W.A. and LaBrie, R.A.: Towards a biochemical classification of depressive disorders I: differences in urinary MHPG and other catecholamine metabolites in clinically defined subtypes of depressions. *Arch. Gen. Psychiatry*, 35:1427-1435, 1978.

53. Schildkraut, J.J., Watson, R., Draskoczy, P.R. and Hartmann, E.: Amphetamine withdrawal: depression and MHPG excretion. *Lancet* *II*:485-486, 1971.

54. Shaskan, E.G. and Becker, R.E.: Platelet monoamine oxidase in schizophrenics. *Nature* 253:659-660, 1975.

55. Shopsin, B., Wilk, S., Gershon, S. Roffman, M. and Goldstein, M.: Collaborative psychopharmacologic studies exploring catecholamine metabolism in psychiatric disorders, In E. Usdin and S. Snyder (Eds.), *Frontiers in Cathecholamine Research*, Pergamon Press, New York, 1973, pp. 173-180.

56. Sullivan, J., Stanfield, C.N. and Dackis, C.: Platelet MAO activity in schizophrenia and other psychiatric illnesses. *Am. J. Psychiatry* 134:1098-1103, 1977.

57. Takahashi, S., Yamane, H. and Tani, H.: Reduction of blood platelet monoamine oxidase activity in schizophrenic patients on phenothiazines. *Folia Psychiat. Neurol. Jpn.* 29:207-214, 1975.

58. Watson, R., Hartmann, E. and Schildkraut, J.J.: Amphetamine withdrawal: affective state, sleep patterns and MHPG excretion. *American J. Psychiatry* 129:263-269, 1972.

59. White, H.L., McLeod, M. and Davidson, J.R.T.: Platelet monoamine oxidase activity in schizophrenia. *Am. J. Psychiatry* 133:1191-1193, 1976.

60. Wilk, S. and Watson, E.: VMA in spinal fluid: evaluation of the pathways of cerebral catecholamine metabolism in man, In. E. Usdin and S. Snyder (Eds.), *Frontiers in Catecholamine Research*, Pergamon Press, New York, 1973, pp. 1067-1069.

61. Wing, J. and Nixon, J.: Discriminating symptoms in schizophrenia. *Arch. Gen. Psychiatry* 32:853-859, 1975.

62. Wyatt, R.J. and Murphy, D. L.: Low platelet monoamine oxidase activity and schizophrenia. *Schizophr. Bull.* 2:77-89, 1976.

63. Wyatt, R.J., Murphy, D.L., Belmaker, R., Cohen, S., Donnelly, C.R.

and Pollin, W.: Reduced monoamine oxidase activity in platelets: a possible genetic marker for vulnerability to schizophrenia. *Science* 173:916-918, 1973.

64. Wyatt, R.J., Potkin, S.G., Gillin, J.C. and Murphy, D.L.: Enzymes involved in phenylethylamine and catecholamine metabolism in schizophrenics and controls, In M. Lipton, A. DiMascio and K. Killam, (Eds.), *Psychopharmacology: A Generation of Progress,* Raven Press, New York, 1978, pp. 1083-1095.

65. Zeller, E.A., Boshes, B., Davis, J.M. and Thorner, M.: Molecular aberration in platelet monoamine oxidase in schizophrenia. *Lancet I*:1385, 1975.

2

New Cellular Mechanisms of Antidepressant Drugs

FRIDOLIN SULSER, M.D.

I. INTRODUCTION

Most of the current hypotheses on the mode of action of antidepressant drugs are based on results derived from pharmacological or biochemical studies involving the interaction of antidepressant drugs with catecholaminergic or serotoninergic mechanisms (46). More recently, tricyclic antidepressants have been shown to be potent competitive inhibitors of the histamine H_2 receptor-mediated response (15) and of the cyclic GMP response mediated by histamine H_1 receptors in cultured mouse neuroblastoma cells (31). Such findings have contributed to the development of animal models of depression and have provided the experimental basis for many screening procedures for the detection of antidepressants as well as for the clinically relevant catecholamine hypothesis of affective disorders. However, hypotheses chiefly derived from studies on acute pharmacological or biochemical effects elicited by antidepressant drugs do not take into consideration the discrepancy in the time course between such effects which occur within minutes and the clinical therapeutic action which requires drug administration for several weeks. Obviously, an acute increase in the availability of catecholamines and/or indolealkylamines is not directly related to the therapeutic efficacy of antidepressant drugs. Moreover, studies with iprindole (11, 20, 35, 36) and mianserin (9, 21) provide evidence that blockade of neuronal reuptake of biogenic amines is not a prerequisite for predicting antidepressant activity in man.

The investigations of this laboratory have been supported by USPHS grants MH-11468, MH-29228 and by the Tennessee Department of Mental Health and Mental Retardation.

Psychotropic Drug Research

While the activity of adrenergic neurons is generally regulatable by intra- and interneuronal feedback mechanisms involving mostly the biosynthesis of catecholamines, studies from our laboratories on functional catecholamine receptor interactions have provided evidence for an additional regulatory mechanism of central noradrenergic neurons at the level of the norepinephrine (NE) receptor coupled adenylate cyclase system (26, 47). It is the aim of this paper to briefly characterize this noradrenergic receptor system in brain and its modification by psychotropic drugs which can either precipitate or alleviate depressive disorders in man.

II. CHARACTERIZATION OF THE NE RECEPTOR COUPLED ADENYLATE CYCLASE SYSTEM IN THE LIMBIC FOREBRAIN

Blumberg et al. (6, 7) have first demonstrated that tissue slices of the rat limbic forebrain incubated in Krebs-Ringer buffer contain a cyclic AMP generating system which is stimulated by low concentrations of NE but not by dopamine or serotonin. This selectivity was of considerable interest because the limbic forebrain receives not only noradrenergic input through the medial forebrain bundle, but dopaminergic fibers originating in the A 10 region and serotoninergic fibers originating in the raphe system also project to this brain area. Since one of the characteristics of a receptor-mediated biological response is the stereospecific activation by agonists, we determined the structure activity relationships and the steric requirements for β-phenylethylamines as agonists of this system. These studies revealed that agonist activity requires a β-3,4 dihydroxyphenethylamine with a β-hydroxy group in the R configuration (Table I). The addition of a N-isopropyl group (isoproterenol) greatly enhances the affinity of an agonist for the cyclic AMP generating system as judged from the EC_{50} value, but markedly decreases the maximal response. Whereas the presence of classical β-receptors in brain is well established, the functional significance of the NE response which is not β in nature remains to be elucidated. Though labelled α-agonists and antagonists bind with high affinity and selectivity to membranes of rat brain (14), classical α-agonists such as phenylephrine, p-hydroxynorephedrine, metaraminol, and methoxamine are devoid of agonist activity in our system, thus indicating that an extrapolation of the α and β receptor concept from the periphery to brain is difficult. It is of interest in this regard that Vetulani et al. (49) demonstrated that the α-agonist phenylephrine actually acts as an NE antagonist.

TABLE I

Effect of various β-phenethylamines on the limbic noradrenergic cyclic AMP generating system.

Compound	R^1	R^2	R^3	R^4	R^5	EC_{50} (μM)	V_{max} % (R)-Norepinephr
(R)-Norepinephrine	OH	OH	OH	H	H	9–11	100
(S)-Norepinephrine	OH	OH	OH	H	H	>245	23 at 1000 μM
(R)-Epinephrine	OH	OH	OH	H	CH₃	7–9	105
(S)-Epinephrine	OH	OH	OH	H	CH₃	>103	79 at 1000 μM
(±)-α-Methylnorepinephrine	OH	OH	OH	CH₃	H	16–20	102
(R)-Isoproterenol	OH	OH	OH	H	CH(CH₃)₂	~0.1	23
(S)-Isoproterenol	OH	OH	OH	H	CH(CH₃)₂	~1.0	20
Dopamine	OH	OH	H	H	H	inactive up to 1000 μM	
(±)-Octopamine	H	OH	OH	H	H	inactive up to 100 μM	
(±)-Phenylephrine	OH	H	OH	H	CH₃	inactive up to 1000 μM	
(S)-Amphetamine	H	H	H	CH₃	H	inactive up to 100 μM	
(R)-Amphetamine	H	H	H	CH₃	H	inactive up to 100 μM	
(S)-p-OH-Amphetamine	H	OH	H	CH₃	H	inactive up to 100 μM	
(R)-p-OH-Amphetamine	H	OH	H	CH₃	H	inactive up to 100 μM	
(αR)-p-OH-Norephedrine	H	OH	OH	CH₃	H	inactive up to 100 μM	
(αS)-p-OH-Norephedrine	H	OH	OH	CH₃	H	inactive up to 100 μM	
(αR)-p-OH-Norpseudophedrine	H	OH	OH	CH₃	H	inactive up to 100 μM	
(αS)-p-OH-Norpseudophedrine	H	OH	OH	CH₃	H	inactive up to 100 μM	
(αS,βR)-Metaraminol	OH	H	OH	CH₃	H	inactive up to 1000 μM	
(±)-Methoxamine	(2,5-diCH₃O)	OH	H	CH₃	H	inactive up to 1000 μM	

The EC_{50} value designates the concentration of agonist that causes a half-maximum response and the V_{max} value the concentration that elicits a maximal increase in the level of cyclic AMP. V_{max} value of (R)-norepinephrine in picomoles cyclic AMP/mg protein ± SEM: 115-1 ± 10.9. From Robinson, S.E., Mobley, P.L., Smith, H.E., and Sulser, F.: Structural and steric requirements for β-phenethylamines as agonists of the noradrenergic cyclic AMP generating system in the rat limbic forebrain. *Naunyn-Schmiedeberg's Arch. Pharmacol.* 303: 175-180, 1978, with permission.

Similar puzzling data with α-agonists have been reported by Skolnick and Daly (40) in cortical slices. The demonstrated lack of additive effects of (R)-NE and (R)-isoproterenol at saturating concentrations (33) seems to exclude the possibility of separate catecholamine receptor coupled adenylate cyclase systems and suggests that isoproterenol activates a subpopulation of adrenergic β-receptors whereas (R)-NE activates at least two populations of adrenergic receptors, one with β-characteristics and the other NE receptors which are not β in nature and which are not stimulated by classical α-agonists. Studies with butaclamol have shown that the neurohormonal response to NE is also stereoselectively blocked by antagonists (32).

The development of supersensitivity following a prolonged reduction in the availability of the agonist is another characteristic of this particular neuronal receptor system. Thus, denervation of limbic forebrain structures by means of electrolytic lesions of the medial forebrain bundle causes an enhanced responsiveness of the adenylate cyclase system to NE (unpublished results). Supersensitivity of the system has also been demonstrated following 6-hydroxydopamine or after subchronic treatment with reserpine (50). This supersensitivity is not associated with a change in the affinity of NE to the receptor, but appears to be the consequence of postsynaptic alteration related to noradrenergic receptor function. An increased responsiveness of this cyclic AMP generating system to NE following 6-hydroxydopamine has also been reported in cortical slices (17, 19, 29, 52) or in slices from the hypothalamus or brain stem (30). It is pertinent that supersensitivity following 6-hydroxydopamine also develops toward isoproterenol which is not taken up by presynaptic nerve terminals (50). The increased β-adrenergic receptor sensitivity in rat cerebral cortex after 6-hydroxydopamine has been shown to be associated with a small increase in the density of β-adrenergic receptor sites (42). The demonstrated supersensitivity of the receptor system might provide the biochemical basis for the observed enhanced behavioral activity following intraventricular NE in animals chemosympathectomized with 6-hydroxydopamine or treated chronically with reserpine (12, 23).

III. DEVELOPMENT OF SUBSENSITIVITY AND DOWN-REGULATION OF β-ADRENERGIC RECEPTORS FOLLOWING ANTIDEPRESSANTS AND ECT

A. MAO Inhibitors

Inhibition of MAO has been linked to an increase in the availability of physiologically active amines at corresponding receptor sites through a spillover from intraneuronal stores. This suggested spillover following inhibition of MAO has been demonstrated to occur in brain *in vivo* (44). It was thus of interest to study the consequences of an increased availability of NE following MAO inhibition on the NE receptor coupled adenylate cyclase system.

Eighteen hours after the administration of a single dose of MAO inhibitors, the cyclic AMP response to NE was markedly enhanced while chronic treatment for three weeks with either pargyline or nialamid significantly reduced the NE response (Figure 1). The

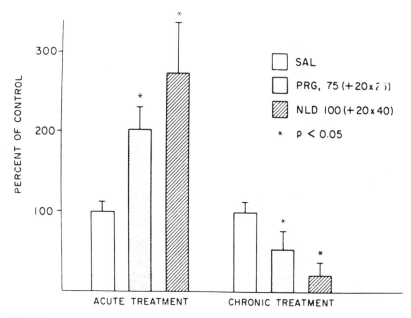

FIGURE 1   Relative cyclic AMP responses to 5 μM NE in slices of the limbic forebrain of rats following acute (single dose) and chronic treatment with MAO inhibitors. Animals were sacrificed 18 hours after the last injection. Pargyline (PRG) was administered at a dose of 75 mg/kg i.p. followed by daily doses of 25 mg/kg i.p. for 20 days. Nialamid (NLD) was given at a dose of 100 mg/kg i.p. followed by daily doses of 40 mg/kg for 20 days. SAL = saline. Control responses to NE in picomoles cyclic AMP/mg protein ± SEM: 47.1 ± 4.9 (N = 18). From Sulser, F. and Vetulani, J.: The noradrenergic cyclic AMP generating system in the limbic forebrain: A functional post-synaptic norepinephrine receptor system and its modification by drugs which either alleviate or precipitate depression. In E. Usdin and I. Hanin, (Eds.), *Models in Psychiatry and Neurology*, Pergamon Press, New York, 189-199, 1977, with permission.

concentration of NE in brain had increased to approximately the same level following a single dose or following chronic administration of the two MAO inhibitors indicating that the change in responsiveness of the system to NE is independent of the concentration of the catecholamine in brain (50). Preliminary results have shown that withdrawal of the MAO inhibitors for nine days resulted in normalization of the cyclic AMP response to NE. The initial shortlived enhanced reactivity of the system to NE is most likely the consequence of a decreased metabolism of NE due to MAO inhibition in a tissue with not yet developed subsensitivity at postsynaptic sites, a process that develops over time.

B. Tricyclic Antidepressants

While a single dose or short term administration of tricyclic antidepressants do not elicit changes in either the basal level or the responsiveness of the cyclic AMP generating system to NE (51), the administration of tricyclic antidepressants on a clinically relevant time basis causes a highly significant reduction in the sensitivity of the NE receptor coupled adenylate cyclase system in the rat limbic forebrain (Table II). This reduction of the neurohormonal response is not related to the concentration of the antidepressant drugs in brain tissue but depends on time (51). The development of subsensitivity of noradrenergic receptors following prolonged treatment with desipramine (DMI) could be the consequence of their chronic overexposure to NE following inhibition of the neuronal reuptake of the catecholamine. The demonstrated subsensitivity to NE following chronic administration of more selective serotonin (5HT) uptake inhibitors such as chlorimipramine and also amitriptyline (25) could be the consequence of the *in vivo* conversion to their corresponding secondary amines, desmethylchlorimipramine and nortriptyline respectively, which are potent inhibitors of the neuronal reuptake of NE. The findings that the most selective 5HT reuptake inhibitor, fluoxetine, and also raphe lesions did not modify the neurohormonal response to NE further support this supposition. However, the subsensitivity developed following chronic administration of iprindole is difficult to understand on this basis, as this drug does not inhibit the neuronal reuptake of NE or alter its metabolism or turnover (11, 20, 35).

The development of subsensitivity of the NE receptor coupled adenylate cyclase system following chronic treatment with tricyclic antidepressants in limbic forebrain and in other brain areas with

TABLE II

Effect of long-term (4-8 weeks) treatment with desipramine or iprindole on the response of the cyclic
AMP generating system in the rat limbic forebrain to NE.

	Time of Sacrifice† (h)	N	Basal Level of Cyclic AMP (pmoles/mg protein ± SEM)	Cyclic AMP Response to NE‡‡ (pmoles/mg protein ± SEM)	Percent of Control Response
Control	1 or 24	15	17.8 ± 2.6	20.4 ± 2.7	100
Desipramine	1	12	20.5 ± 2.7	9.9 ± 3.5*	49
Desipramine	24	14	16.6 ± 1.6	6.9 ± 2.1***	34
Iprindole	1	13	22.3 ± 3.6	9.4 ± 4.7*	46
Iprindole	24	15	16.9 ± 1.5	7.9 ± 2.4**	38

* $p < 0.05$; ** $p < 0.01$; *** $p < 0.001$ (difference from control response; Student t-test).
† Time after last injection.
‡‡ Difference in the level of cyclic AMP between the preparation exposed to 5 μM NE and that of the control preparation (corre-
sponding hemisection).
From Vetulani, J., Stawarz, R.J., Dingell, J.V. and Sulser, F.: A possible common mechanism of action of antidepressant treatments. *Naunyn-Schmiedeberg's Arch. Pharmacol.* 293:109-114, 1976, with permission.

noradrenergic projections has been confirmed in a number of laboratories (10, 37, 38). Tricyclic antidepressants thus share this delayed action on the NE receptor coupled adenylate system (regardless of their action at presynaptic sites) with MAO inhibitor-type antidepressants.

Recent *in vivo* studies have provided additional evidence for a down-regulation of central adrenergic activity following chronic administration of tricyclic antidepressants. Thus, a reduced *in vivo* accumulation of cyclic AMP occurs in rat cerebral cortex following stimulation of the locus coeruleus in animals treated chronically with tricyclic antidepressants (18). Moreover, while acute treatment with DMI enhances the inhibitory effect of NE on cerebellar Purkinje firing, chronic treatment with the antidepressant inhibits the effect of NE on the firing rate.*

C. Amphetamine–like Drugs

The rather poor therapeutic response to amphetamine in depression is surprising as this phenylethylamine derivative shares pharmacologic properties with both MAO inhibitors and tricyclic antidepressants and thus should increase the availability of NE at postsynaptic receptor sites. Recent results by Mobley *et al.* (27) have shown that chronic administration of high doses of amphetamine can cause subsensitivity of the limbic cyclic AMP generating system to NE thus confirming data obtained by Baudry et al. (3) in mice and by Stone (43) in cortical slices of the rat. Amphetamine, even in high doses is, however, a rather weak desensitizer of the system affecting predominantly the maximal response to NE and not the affinity of NE to the receptor system. However, if the aromatic hydroxylation of amphetamine is inhibited by iprindole, amphetamine causes a very rapid and pronounced state of subsensitivity of the receptor coupled adenylate cyclase system to NE (Figure 2) and isoproterenol (13). The rather poor response to amphetamine appears to be the consequence of its short biological half-life (approximately 45 minutes) and possibly of the accumulation in noradrenergic neurons of its metabolite (αS, βR)-p-hydroxynorephedrine, a partial NE antagonist, both of which would tend to reduce a persistent agonist receptor interaction (27).

D. Electroconvulsive Treatment (ECT)

ECT is one of the most effective treatments in severe depression

*Bloom, F.E., FASEB Meeting, Atlantic City, 1978.

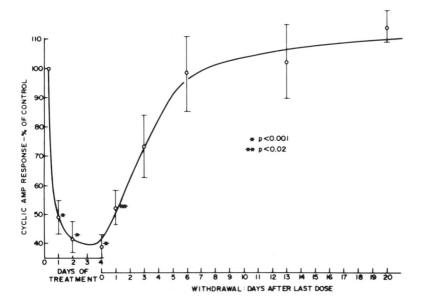

FIGURE 2   Cyclic AMP responses to 10 μM NE following inhibition of the aromatic hydroxylation of amphetamine by iprindole. Iprindole was administered i.p. (10 mg/kg/day) followed by amphetamine (10 mg/kg b.i.d.). The results are expressed as a percentage of the corresponding cyclic AMP response to NE in animals treated with saline (control response). From Manier, D.H., Gillespie, D.D. and Sulser, F.: Effect of (S)-amphetamine on limbic cyclic AMP responses to (R)-norepinephrine following inhibition of aromatic hydroxylation by iprindole. *Fed. Proc.* 37:699, 1978, with permission.

and the onset of its therapeutic action is generally considered to be more rapid than that of pharmacotherapy. Since ECT has been shown to increase the turnover of NE in brain (5) and to decrease the high affinity uptake of the catecholamine (16), it was of interest to study the effect of this clinically effective nondrug treatment on the NE receptor coupled adenylate cyclase system. The daily administration of ECT for eight days caused an approximately 50% reduction in the cyclic AMP response to NE and this reduced responsiveness was still apparent seven days following cessation of ECT (51). Since part of the NE response is β in nature, it is of interest that ECT induces also rapid subsensitivity to the β-adrenergic agonist isoproterenol in both limbic forebrain and frontal cortex (Table III).

37

TABLE III

Effect of electroconvulsive treatment (ECT) on cyclic AMP responses to norepinephrine or isoproterenol in rat limbic forebrain and frontal cortex.

	Limbic Forebrain		Frontal Cortex	
	Response* pmoles/mg protein ± SEM	Percent of Control Response	Response* pmoles/mg protein ± SEM	Percent of Control Response
Norepinephrine (300 µM)				
Control	131.81 ± 11.63 (8)	100	48.48 ± 9.92 (6)	100
ECT	82.88 ± 2.32 (8)†††	63†††	20.41 ± 3.07 (8)†	42†
Isoproterenol (10 µM)				
Control	65.00 ± 5.38 (8)	100	68.75 ± 5.70 (8)	100
ECT	48.14 ± 3.84 (8)†	74†	36.80 ± 5.93 (8)††	53††

ECT was applied b.i.d. for 3 days by passing a current (100 mA; 300 ms) through ear clip electrodes. Control animals had the electrodes attached but no current was passed. The animals were decapitated 18 hours after the last treatment.

*Difference of level in cyclic AMP between the preparation exposed to norepinephrine or isoproterenol and the non-exposed preparation (Basal level). Basal levels in pmoles/mg protein ± SEM: Limbic forebrain, 15.23 ± 2.49 (4) in the absence and 42.12 ± 2.77 (4) in the presence of the phosphodiesterase inhibitor RO 20-1724; Cortex 26.01 ± 4.65 (4) in the absence and 57.41 ± 6.75 (4) in the presence of the phosphodiesterase inhibitor RO 20-1724. Values represent the means of two experiments, each determined in quadruplicate or triplicate. Numbers in parentheses indicate the number of samples. † p < 0.02; †† p < 0.01; ††† p < 0.001. (Gillespie, D.D., Manier, D.H. and Sulser, F., unpublished results from the laboratory).

Antidepressant Drugs

IV. MOLECULAR BASIS OF CHANGES IN SENSITIVITY OF THE NE RECEPTOR COUPLED ADENYLATE CYCLASE SYSTEM BY PSYCHOTROPIC DRUGS

Sensitivity changes by drugs of the NE receptor coupled adenylate cyclase system may occur by changing the affinity of the agonist to the receptor, changing the number or conformation of receptors in the phospholipid membrane, changing the coupling of the occupied receptor to adenylate cyclase, changing the catalytic activity of adenylate cyclase, or the activity of phosphodiesterase. With regard to the β-adrenergic receptor coupled adenylate cyclase in nonneuronal tissue, considerable evidence supports the view that the β-adrenergic receptor and adenylate cyclase are distinct molecular entitites. For example, when β-adrenergic receptors and adenylate cyclase in frog erythrocyte membranes were solubilized and then chromatographed on an agarose 6 B column, both the β-adrenergic receptor binding sites (assayed by specific ^{3}H-dihydroalprenolol binding) and the enzyme adenylate cyclase (preactivated with guanine nucleotides) emerged with very distinct elution profiles (Figure 3).

Although it has not yet been possible to label with certainty central NE receptors which are not β in nature and not stimulated by α-agonists, the direct identification and characterization of β-adrenergic receptors in brain has been possible. Using either ^{3}H-dihydroalprenolol (DHA) or ^{125}I-hydroxybenzylpindolol (HBP) as ligands, the density of β-adrenergic receptors in various brain regions is surprisingly homogenous (1, 8, 41). Using DHA or HBP of high specific activity as ligands of β-adrenergic receptors in brain, it has been demonstrated that supersensitivity or subsensitivity of the NE receptor coupled adenylate cyclase system are linked to a change in the specific labelling of β-adrenergic receptor sites. Thus, the supersensitivity to NE and isoproterenol elicited by 6-hydroxydopamine is associated with an increase in the concentration of HBP binding sites in the cortex of rats without a change in the K_D value of HBP (42). The subsensitivity of the NE receptor coupled adenylate cyclase system following chronic treatment with tricyclic antidepressants is associated with a decrease in the specific ^{3}H-DHA binding (Table IV). Scatchard analysis of such data (Table V) indicates that the principal effect of chronic treatment with tricyclic antidepressants is a reduction in the density of β-adrenergic receptors without a change in the binding affinity or K_D value (2, 4, 39). Since binding characteristics of α-antagonists e.g., ^{3}H-dihydro-

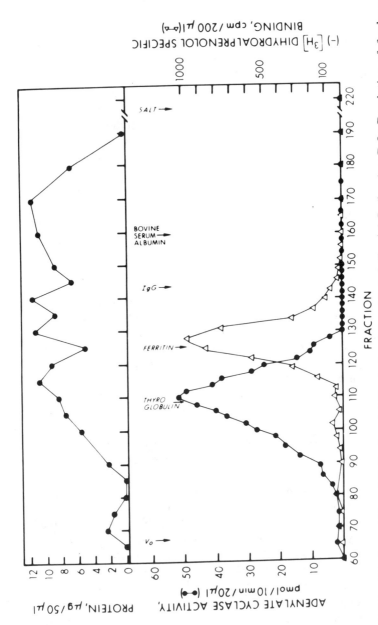

FIGURE 3 Elution profiles of digitonin-solubilized adenylate cyclase and β-adrenergic receptors. Frog erythrocyte membranes, pretreated with 10^{-4} M Gpp(NH)p, were solubilized with 0.6% digitonin, concentrated by Amicon ultra filtration and chromatographed on a Sepharose 6B column. From Lim- bird, L.E. and Lefkowitz, R.J.: Resolution of β-adrenergic receptor and adenylate cyclase activity by gel exclusion chromatography. *J. Biol. Chem.* 252:799-802, 1977, with permission.

Antidepressant Drugs

TABLE IV

Effect of chronic administration of antidepressants
on specific dihydroalprenolol binding.

Drug Treatment	Specific ^{3}H-dihydroalprenolol Binding pmoles/mg protein ± SEM	
	Cortex	Limbic Forebrain
None	0.252 ± 0.016	0.295 ± 0.025
Desipramine (DMI)	0.163 ± 0.019*	0.226 ± 0.015**
Iprindole	0.196 ± 0.020**	0.199 ± 0.015*

Desipramine or iprindole (20 mg/kg i.p.) were administered daily for a period of 2 weeks. Direct labelling of β-adrenergic receptor sites was carried out essentially according to Bylund and Snyder (8). Specific binding is defined as the difference in bound ligand in the presence and absence of 100 μM (±)-propranolol. (Mobley, P.L. unpublished data from this laboratory).

* p < 0.01
** p < 0.05

TABLE V

Scatchard analysis of specific ^{3}H-dihydroalprenolol binding to brains of control and chronically desipramine-treated rats.

	Dissociation Constant (nM)	Density of Receptors (pmoles/mg protein)
Control	0.82 ± 0.08	95 ± 5
DMI (10 mg/kg/day for 6 weeks)	1.09 ± 0.14	59 ± 3*

* p < 0.001.
From Banerjee, L.P., Kung, L.S., Riggi, S.T. and Chanda, S.K.: Development of β-adrenergic receptor subsensitivity by antidepressants. *Nature* 268:455-456, 1977, with permission.

ergocryptine or of ^{3}H-serotonin were not altered following chronic treatment with antidepressants (4, 55), the data indicate that these drugs selectively reduce the number of β-adrenergic receptors. Recent results indicate that the ECT induced subsensitivity of the NE receptor coupled adenylate cyclase system is also linked to a significant decrease in the number of β-adrenergic receptor sites without a change in the K_D value.* As in other systems, the increase (reserpine, 6-hydroxydopamine) or fall (MAO inhibitors, tricyclic

*Gillespie, D.D., Manier, D.H. and Sulser, F., Unpublished results from this laboratory.

antidepressants, ECT) in the number of functional β-adrenergic receptor binding sites (as assayed by antagonist binding) has been of much lower magnitude than the enhancement (supersensitivity) or decrement (subsensitivity) in the NE or isoproterenol stimulated adenylate cyclase activity. This discrepancy may, however, be more apparent than real because catecholamine sensitive adenylate cyclase activity is a function of agonist binding whereas the density of β-adrenergic receptors is inferred from antagonist binding to supersensitive or subsensitive receptor systems. Indeed, following β-adrenergic receptor desensitization, Wessels, *et al.* (53) have demonstrated a close agreement between the reduction in agonist binding (^{3}H-hydroxybenzylisoproterenol) and in hormone stimulated adenylate cyclase activity in membrane fractions derived from frog erythrocytes, whereas binding of the β-adrenergic antagonist ^{3}H-DHA was significantly less affected by desensitization.

While the bulk of data obtained in either peripheral systems or in brain indicates that the down-regulation of β-adrenergic receptors is agonist-specific and depends on the supply of ligand, a change in the availability of agonists to the receptor appears, however, not to be the only mechanism by which either the sensitivity to NE or the number of adrenergic receptors are regulated (Table VI). Thus, iprindole which does not inhibit neuronal reuptake of NE, also decreases both the sensitivity of the system to NE and the density of β-adrenergic receptors (2, 51) and nisoxetine, a potent inhibitor of NE reuptake, does not change the sensitivity of the NE receptor coupled adenylate cyclase system, at least not in tissue slices of the limbic forebrain (37). At this time, one can only speculate

TABLE VI

Drug induced changes in the availability of NE and regulation of the NE receptor coupled adenylate cyclase system.

	DMI	Iprindole	Nisoxetine
Availability of NE at Receptor	↑↑↑	0	↑↑↑
Sensitivity of the NE Receptor Coupled Adenylate Cyclase System	↓↓↓	↓↓↓	0*
Density of β-Adrenergic Receptors	↓↓↓	↓↓↓	?
Tyrosine Hydroxylase Activity	↓↓↓	↓↓↓	?

↑↑↑ increase; ↓↓↓ decrease; 0 no change.
*Schmidt and Thornberry (37).

about the fate of neuronal β-adrenergic receptors which can no longer be detected by radiolabelled β-adrenergic ligands. The elucidation of the probably multiple mechanisms involved in the loss or acquisition of binding sites as well as the mechanisms involved in coupling of the occupied receptor to adenylate cyclase within the phospholipid matrix of neuronal membranes remain exciting areas for future research.

V. PHARMACOLOGICAL DISTINCTION BETWEEN DESENSITIZATION AND BLOCKADE OF THE NE RECEPTOR COUPLED ADENYLATE CYCLASE SYSTEM

With regards to adrenergic blocking properties, there exist similarities in the pharmacologic and biochemical profile between tertiary amines of tricyclic antidepressants and chlorpromazine-like antipsychotic drugs. However, the tertiary amines of tricyclic antidepressants are converted *in vivo* to their corresponding secondary amines which through blockade of NE reuptake cause initially an enhancement of adrenergic activity followed by a delayed subsensitivity of the NE receptor coupled adenylate cyclase systems linked to a down-regulation of β-adrenergic receptors. The antipsychotic drug chlorpromazine causes also desensitization of the NE receptor coupled adenylate cyclase system (38), probably as a consequence of presynaptic α-blockade and blockade of neuronal reuptake of NE, both of which would tend to increase the availability of NE at its receptor sites. Despite these overlaps in pharmacological activity, the overall synaptic dynamics for adrenergic receptor blockers and drugs which cause predominantly subsensitivity of the receptor system following their chronic administration are quite different (Table VII). It is conceivable that these subtle differences in pharmacological activity elicited at the level of adrenergic receptors may determine to a great degree the clinical profile of the drug, that is, whether a drug is useful for the treatment of schizophrenia (antipsychotic drugs) or for the alleviation of predominantly affective disorders (MAO inhibitors, tricyclic antidepressants, and ECT).

VI. FUNCTIONAL SIGNIFICANCE OF SENSITIVITY CHANGES OF THE NE RECEPTOR COUPLED ADENYLATE CYCLASE SYSTEM IN BRAIN

The findings that psychotropic drugs which either can precipitate (e.g., reserpine) or alleviate (MAO inhibitors, tricyclic antidepres-

TABLE VII

Pharmacological distinction between blockade and desensitization of central noradrenergic receptor function by psychotropic drugs.

Central NE-Receptor Blockade by Drug	Desensitization of Central NE-Receptor Coupled Cyclic AMP Generating System by Drug
1. Blockade is easily demonstrated *in vitro*	1. No blockade *in vitro* (in reasonable molar concentrations)
2. Blockade depends on concentration of drug in tissue	2. Desensitization is not dependent on concentration of drug in tissue but instead depends on time
3. No change in density of β-adrenergic receptors	3. Desensitization is linked to down-regulation of β-adrenergic receptors
4. Drug activates interneuronal feedback mechanisms: a. Increase in the activity of tyrosine hydroxylase b. Increase in the rate of turnover of catecholamines	4. Drug does not activate interneuronal feedback mechanisms: a. No increase in the activity of tyrosine hydroxylase b. No increase in the rate of turnover of catecholamines
5. Usually, drug also blocks markedly DA receptors	5. No blockade of DA receptors

Adapted from Sulser, F. and Robinson, S.E.: Clinical implications of pharmacological differences among antipsychotic drugs (with particular emphasis on biochemical central synaptic adrenergic mechanisms), In, M.A. Lipton, A. DiMascio and K.F. Killam, (Eds.), *Psychopharmacology: A generation of Progress*, Raven Press, New York, pp. 943-954, 1978, with permission.

TABLE VIII

Summary of effects of psychotropic drugs on turnover of norepinephrine and on norepinephrine receptor mediated cyclic AMP responses.

Agent	Effect on Turnover of Brain NE	Responsiveness of Nor-adrenergic Cyclic AMP Generating System to NE	Clinical Therapeutic Action
Reserpine	↑↑↑	↑↑↑	Precipitates depression in man
6-OHDA	↓↓↓	↑↑↑	Precipitates "depression" in monkeys
MAO-inhibitors	↓↓↓	↓↓↓	Antidepressant
Imipramine-like drugs (following chronic administration)	↑↑↑* ↓↓↓**	↓↓↓	Antidepressant
Iprindole	0	↓↓↓	Antidepressant
ECT	↑↑↑	↓↓↓	Antidepressant

↑↑↑ increased; ↓↓↓ decreased; 0 no effect.
* Roffman et al. (34).
** Nielsen and Braestrup (28).
From Sulser, F.: Functional aspects of the norepinephrine receptor coupled adenylate cyclase system in the limbic forebrain and its modification by drugs which precipitate or alleviate depression: Molecular approaches to an understanding of affective disorders, *Pharmakopsychiatrie* 11: 43-52, 1978, with permission.

sants, and ECT) depressive illness change the sensitivity of the NE receptor coupled adenylate cyclase system in opposite directions (supersensitivity or subsensitivity, respectively) should provide a new theoretical framework for studies on the psychobiology of depression. In comparing the acute pharmacological actions of antidepressant treatments on presynaptic sites (e.g., NE turnover) with those elicited on NE receptor mediated events following treatment on a clinically relevant time basis (Table VIII), it becomes evident that the delayed therapeutic action is better related to the delayed changes occurring at the level of the NE receptor coupled adenylate cyclase system than to acute changes at presynaptic sites. The precise role of the linked reduction in the density of β-adrenergic receptors in the molecular mechanism of neuronal receptor subsensitivity to NE is not yet known. It is most likely that the change in the number of functional β-receptors is only one aspect by which the sensitivity of the NE receptor coupled adenylate cyclase-protein kinase system in brain and thus the kinetic amplification of the noradrenergic cyclic AMP mediated information flow are regulated. In any event, the exploration of the neurobiological consequences of a change in this information flow can now be experimentally approached and new methodology to elucidate the substrates of protein kinase *in vivo* is certainly forthcoming.

Extrapolated to the clinical situation, one is tempted to advance the hypothesis that depression prone patients may suffer from an inability to regulate the noradrenergic cyclic AMP protein kinase mediated information flow and that successful treatment with antidepressants or ECT depends on the successful desensitization of the NE receptor coupled adenylate cyclase system, thus causing a reduction in the postulated amplification mechanism involved in e.g., the regulation of arousal and internal affective states. In this regard, it is noteworthy that neurophysiological studies in patients with affective disorders indicate that central hyperarousal is a prominent characteristic of both depressive and manic states (54). Certainly, as our understanding of molecular events at postsynaptic sites deepens, new and exciting possibilities arise at the horizon for the development of more specific psychotropic drugs.

REFERENCES

1. Alexander, R.W., Davis, J.N. and Lefkowitz, R.J.: Direct identification and characterization of β-adrenergic receptors in rat brain. *Nature* 258:437-440, 1975.

2. Banerjee, L.P., Kung, L.S., Riggi, S.T. and Chanda, S.K.: Development of β-adrenergic receptor subsensitivity by antidepressants. *Nature* 268:455-456, 1977.
3. Baudry, M., Martres, M.P. and Schwartz, J.C.: Modulation in the sensitivity of noradrenergic receptors in the CNS studied by the responsiveness of the cyclic AMP system. *Brain Res.* 116:111-124, 1976.
4. Bergstrom, D.A., Bortz, R.J. and Kellar, K.J.: Adrenergic and serotonergic receptor binding in brain after chronic desipramine (DMI) treatment. *Fed. Proc.* 37:1939, 1978.
5. Bliss, E.L., Ailison, T. and Zwanziger, J.: Metabolism of norepinephrine, serotonin and dopamine in rat brain with stress. *J. Pharmacol. Exp. Ther.* 164:122-134, 1968.
6. Blumberg, J.B., Taylor, R.E. and Sulser, F.: Blockade by pimozide of norepinephrine-sensitive adenylate cyclase in the limbic forebrain: Possible role of limbic noradrenergic mechanisms in the mode of action of antipsychotics. *J. Pharm. Pharmacol.* 27:125-128, 1975.
7. Blumberg, J.B., Vetulani, J., Stawarz, R.J. and Sulser, F.: The noradrenergic cyclic AMP generating system in the limbic forebrain: Pharmacological characterization and possible role of limbic noradrenergic mechanism in the mode of action of antipsychotic drugs. *Europ. J. Pharmacol.* 37:357-366, 1976.
8. Bylund, D.B. and Snyder, S.H.: Beta-adrenergic receptor binding in membrane preparations from mammalian brain. *Mol. Pharmacol.* 12:568-580, 1976.
9. Coppen, A., Ghose, K., Swade, C. and Wood, K.: Effect of mianserin hydrochloride on peripheral uptake mechanisms for noradrenaline and 5-hydroxytryptamine in man. *Br. J. Clin. Pharmacol.* 5:135-185, 1978.
10. Frazer, A. and Mendels, J.: Do tricyclic antidepressants enhance adrenergic transmission? *Am. J. Psychiatry* 134:1040-1042, 1977.
11. Freeman, J.J. and Sulser, F.: Iprindole-amphetamine interactions in the rat: The role of aromatic hydroxylation of amphetamine in its mode of action. *J. Pharmacol. Exp. Ther.* 183:307-315, 1972.
12. Geyer, M.A. and Segal, D.S.: Differential effects of reserpine and α-methyl-p-tyrosine on norepinephrine and dopamine induced behavioral activity. *Psychopharmacologia* 29:131-138, 1973.
13. Gillespie, D.D., Manier, D.H. and Sulser, F.: Normalization by amphetamine of the reserpine induced hypersensitivity of the noradrenergic cyclic AMP generating system in brain. *Pharmacologist* 20:430, 1978.
14. Greenberg, D.A., U'Prichard, D.C. and Snyder, S.H.: Alpha-noradrenergic receptor binding in mammalian brain: Differential labelling of agonist and antagonist states. *Life Sci.* 19:69-76, 1976.
15. Green, J.P. and Maayani, S.: Tricyclic antidepressant drugs block histamine H_2 receptor in brain. *Nature* 269:163-165, 1977.
16. Hendley, E.D. and Welch, B.L.: Electroconvulsive shock: Sustained decrease in norepinephrine uptake in a reserpine model of depression.

Life Sci. 16:45-54, 1975.

17. Huang, M., Ho, A.K.S. and Daly, J.W.: Accumulation of adenosine 3', 5'-monophosphate in rat cerebral cortical slices. *Mol. Pharmacol.* 9: 711-717, 1973.

18. Korf, J., Sebens, J.B. and Postema, F.: Cyclic AMP in the rat cerebral cortex: Role of the locus coeruleus and effects of antidepressants. *Abstracts 7th Internat. Cong. Pharmacol.*, Paris, France, Abstract 291, 1978.

19. Kalisker, A., Rutledge, C.H.O. and Perkins, J.P.: Effect of nerve degeneration by 6-hydroxydopamine on catecholamine-stimulated adenosine 3',5'-monophosphate formation in rat cerebral cortex. *Mol. Pharmacol.* 9:619-629, 1973.

20. Lahti, R.A. and Maickel, R.P.: The tricyclic antidepressants —inhibition of norepinephrine uptake as related to potentiation of norepinephrine and clinical efficacy. *Biochem. Pharmacol.* 20:482-486, 1971.

21. Leonard, B.E.: Some effects of mianserin on monoamine metabolism in the rat brain. *Br. J. Clin. Pharmacol.* 5:115-125, 1978.

22. Limbird, L.E. and Lefkowitz, R.J.: Resolution of β-adrenergic receptor and adenylate cyclase activity by gel exclusion chromatography. *J. Biol. Chem.* 252:799-802, 1977.

23. Mandell, A.J.: The role of adaptive regulation in the pathophysiology of psychiatric disease. *J. Psychiatry Res.* 11:173-179, 1974.

24. Manier, D.H., Gillespie, D.D. and Sulser, F.: Effect of (S)-amphetamine on limbic cyclic AMP responses to (R)-norepinephrine following inhibition of aromatic hydroxylation by iprindole. *Fed. Proc.* 37:699, 1978.

25. Mishra, R. and Sulser, F.: Role of serotonin reuptake inhibition in the development of subsensitivity of the norepinephrine (NE) receptor coupled adenylate cyclase system. *Comm. Psychopharmacol.*, 2: 365-370, 1978.

26. Mobley, P.L., Mishra, R. and Sulser, F.: Characterization, adaptation and regulatory changes of the norepinephrine (NE) receptor coupled adenylate cyclase system in limbic forebrain structures, In E. Usdin and J. Barchas (Eds.): *Catecholamines: Basic and Clinical Frontiers,* Pergamon Press, New York, 1979, pp. 523-525.

27. Mobley, P.L., Sanders-Bush, E., Smith, H.E. and Sulser, F.: Modification of the noradrenergic cyclic AMP generating system in the rat limbic forebrain by amphetamine: Role of its hydroxylated metabolites. *Naunyn-Schmiedeberg's Arch. Pharmacol.*, 306:267-273, 1979.

28. Nielsen, M. and Braestrup, C.: Chronic treatment with desipramine caused a sustained decrease of 3,4-dihydroxyphenylglycol-sulfate and total 3-methoxy-4-hydroxy phenylglycol in the rat brain. *Naunyn-Schmiedeberg's Arch. Pharmacol.* 300:87-92, 1977.

29. Palmer, G.C.: Increased cyclic AMP response to norepinephrine in the rat brain following 6-hydroxydopamine. *Neuropharmacology* 11:145-149, 1972.

30. Palmer, G.C., Sulser, F. and Robison, G.A.: Effect of neurohumoral and adrenergic agents on cyclic AMP levels in various areas of the rat brain *in vitro. Neuropharmacology* 12:327-338, 1973.

31. Richelson, E.: Histamine H_1 receptor mediated guanosine 3',5'-monophosphate formation by cultured mouse neuroblastoma cells. *Science* 201:69-71, 1978.

32. Robinson, S.E. and Sulser, F.: The noradrenergic cyclic AMP generating system of the rat limbic forebrain and its stereospecificity for (+) butaclamol. *J. Pharm. Pharmacol.* 28:645-646, 1976.

33. Robinson, S.E., Mobley, P.L., Smith, H.E. and Sulser, F.: Structural and steric requirements for β-phenethylamines as agonists of the noradrenergic cyclic AMP generating system in the rat limbic forebrain. *Naunyn-Schmiedeberg's Arch. Pharmacol.* 303:175-180, 1978.

34. Roffman, M., Kling, A., Cassens, G., Orsulak, P.J., Reigle, T.G. and Schildkraut, J.J.: The effects of acute and chronic administration of tricyclic antidepressants on $MHPG\text{-}SO_4$ in rat brain. *Comm. Psychopharmacol.* 1:195-206, 1977.

35. Rosloff, B.N. and Davis, J.M.: Effect of iprindole on norepinephrine turnover and transport. *Psychopharmacologia* 40:53-64, 1974.

36. Sanghvi, I. and Gershon, S.: Effect of acute and chronic iprindole on serotonin turnover in mouse brain. *Biochem. Pharmacol.* 24:2103-2104, 1975.

37. Schmidt, M.J. and Thornberry, J.F.: Norepinephrine-stimulated cyclic AMP accumulation in brain slices *in vitro* after serotonin depletion or chronic administration of selective amine reuptake inhibitors. *Arch. Int. Pharmacodyn.* 229:42-51, 1977.

38. Schultz, J.: Psychoactive drug effects on a system which generates cyclic AMP in brain. *Nature* 261:417-418, 1976.

39. Sellinger, M., Sarai, K., Frazer, A., Mendels, J. and Hess, M.E.: Beta-adrenergic receptor binding in rat cerebral cortex after repeated administration of psychotropic drugs. *Fed. Proc.* 37:518, 1978.

40. Skolnick, P. and Daly, J.W.: Stimulation of adenosine 3',5'-monophosphate formation by α- and β-adrenergic agonists in rat cerebral cortical slices: Effect of clonidine. *Molec. Pharmacol.* 11:545-551, 1975.

41. Sporn, J.R. and Molinoff, P.B.: Beta adrenergic receptors in rat brain. *J. Cyclic Nucl. Res.* 2:149-161, 1976.

42. Sporn, J.R., Harden, T.K., Wolfe, B.B. and Molinoff, P.B.: β-Adrenergic receptor involvement in 6-hydroxydopamine induced supersensitivity in rat cerebral cortex. *Science* 194:624-626, 1976.

43. Stone, E.A.: Effect of stress on norepinephrine stimulated cyclic AMP formation in brain slices, *Pharmacol. Biochem. Behav.* 8:583-591, 1978.

44. Strada, S.J. and Sulser, F.: Effect of monoamine oxidase inhibitors on metabolism and *in vivo* release of H^3-norepinephrine from the hypothalamus. *Europ. J. Pharmacol.* 18:303-308, 1972.

45. Sulser, F. and Robinson, S.E.: Clinical implications of pharmacological

differences among antipsychotic drugs (with particular emphasis on biochemical central synaptic adrenergic mechanisms), In M. A. Lipton, A. DiMascio and K.F. Killam, (Eds.), *Psychopharmacology: A Generation of Progress*, Raven Press, New York, pp. 943-954, 1978.

46. Sulser, F.: Tricyclic antidepressants: Animal pharmacology (Biochemical and metabolic aspects), In L.L. Iverson, S.D. Iversen, and S.H. Snyder, (Eds.), *Handbook of Psychopharmacology*, Volume 14, Plenum Press, New York, pp. 157-197, 1978.

47. Sulser, F.: Functional aspects of the norepinephrine receptor coupled adenylate cyclase system in the limbic forebrain and its modification by drugs which precipitate or alleviate depression: Molecular approaches to an understanding of affective disorders, *Pharmakopsychiatrie* 11:43-52, 1978.

48. Sulser, F. and Vetulani, J.: The noradrenergic cyclic AMP generating system in the limbic forebrain: A functional post-synaptic norepinephrine receptor system and its modification by drugs which either alleviate or precipitate depression. In E. Usdin and I. Hanin, (Eds.), *Models in Psychiatry and Neurology*, Pergamon Press, New York, 189-199, 1977.

49. Vetulani, J., Leith, N.J., Stawarz, R.J. and Sulser, F.: Effect of clonidine on the noradrenergic cyclic AMP generating system in the limbic forebrain and on medial forebrain self-stimulation behavior. *Experientia* 33:1490-1492, 1977.

50. Vetulani, J., Stawarz, R.J. and Sulser, F.: Adaptive mechanisms of the noradrenergic cyclic AMP generating system in the limbic forebrain of the rat: Adaptation to persistent changes in the availability of norepinephrine (NE). *J. Neurochem.* 27:661-666, 1976.

51. Vetulani, J., Stawarz, R.J., Dingell, J.V. and Sulser, F.: A possible common mechanism of action of antidepressant treatments. *Naunyn-Schmiedeberg's Arch. Pharmacol.* 293:109-114, 1976.

52. Weiss, B. and Strada, S.: Neuroendocrine control of the cyclic AMP system of brain and pineal gland. *Adv. Cyclic Nucl. Res.* 1:357-374, 1972.

53. Wessels, M.R., Mullikin, D. and Lefkowitz, R.J.: Differences between agonist and antagonist binding following β-adrenergic receptor desensitization. *J. Biol. Chem.* 253:3371-3373, 1978.

54. Whybrow, P. and Mendels, J.: Toward a biology of depression: Some suggestions from neurophysiology. *Am. J. Psychiatry* 125:45-54, 1969.

55. Wirz-Justice, A., Krauchi, K., Lichtsteiner, M. and Feer, H.: Is it possible to modify serotonin receptor sensitivity? *Life Sci.* 280:1249-1254, 1978.

3

Future Drugs against Senescence-Related Brain Dysfunction

HARBANS LAL, Ph.D. and
KALIDAS NANDY, M.D., Ph.D.

I. ELDERLY POPULATION AND PHARMACEUTICAL NEEDS

It is very significant that the editors of this monograph consider future drug development of geriatric applications to be important. Usually drug developers ignore the elderly. Perhaps what has compelled the present editors to be unusual is the alarming prospects of the impact that our aging population will soon make on the American society and the health care industry. Recent surveys show that the number of people over 65 years of age in the United States is increasing at the annual rate of nearly 400,000 making this the most rapidly expanding segment of our population. It is estimated that by the year 2000 there will be nearly 30 million elderly Americans as consumers of our pharmaceutical services. It is also estimated that the elderly use 2.2 times more drugs than their younger counterpart so that drugs employed by the elderly will be equivalent to those usually consumed by a population of 67 million. Besides, there are new indications that estimates on the rate of increase in the elderly may have to be revised in the future because of the expected progress in medicine and health service that will lead to reduction of mortality. For instance, the extensive efforts devoted to the search for more effective measures for prevention and treatment of heart disease, malignant neoplasia, and cerebrovascular diseases, which together account for three out of every four deaths in the United States (25), will certainly augment the usual increase in the elderly population.

Based upon an invited lecture presented by Dr. H. Lal at H-RPI Symposium on New Frontiers of Psychotropic Drug Development, Hershey, Pa., Oct. 17-19, 1978.

Psychotropic Drug Research

Of great significance is the fact that the population of elderly persons who survive beyond the age of 75 is continually increasing. This group is expected to account for 43% of the total elderly population in 2000. An important characteristic of this group of the aged that is most burdensome is the occurrence of a mental disorder commonly known as dementia. Of all the geriatric patients that are admitted to long-term institutional care, 62% are dementia. Patients with dementia usually require intensive personal as well as medical care which often constitutes a burden to families, to health professionals, to service facilities, to the tax payers, and to society as a whole. This is so because occurrence of dementia is incompatible with self-help and our ability to treat dementia is presently very limited. It is proposed that new frontiers of research should aim at the development of drugs that are active in preventing the onset of dementia and those active in treating the dementia after its onset. The approach taken should be multidisciplinary so that several different aspects of the new findings can be correlated to produce reliable leads for clinical application. It is attempted here to briefly review the neuropathological and neurochemical changes that occur in the aged with emphasis on those changes which can be corrected with the present know-how in drug development. A number of experimental models and protocols will be proposed for the benefit of those who are considering entering this field of research.

It must be pointed out right in the beginning that geriatric neuropathology is in its infancy as a scientific discipline. Most known observations have been superficial and derived from subjects suffering from a number of pathological conditions. It is only recently that some investigators have begun to undertake systematic research on the age-related changes in normal animals and human subjects.

II. MORPHOLOGICAL ALTERATIONS IN THE AGING BRAIN

The brain has been the focus of geriatric studies for many years. There are three reasons for its central importance in this respect. First of all, the brain is the controlling organ for mental functions that deteriorate in the aged. Secondly, its functional and structural units are very susceptible to aging. Thirdly, the brain controls most of the endocrine functions that control many metabolic processes essential to the normal working of the body physiology.

The neuropathological changes reported to be found in senescence

Future Drugs against Senescence

TABLE I
Neuropathological changes in the brain related to senescence.

Gross Changes

    Reduction of brain weight
    Reduction of brain volume
    Increase in ventricular size
    Increase in size of sulci

Microscopic Changes

    Loss of neurons
    Deposition of lipofuscin pigments
    Loss of dendritic spines
    Amyloid lesions
    Senile (neuritic) plaques
    Formation of neurofibrillary tangles

Neurophysiological and Behavioral Changes

    Impairment of cognitive functions
    Impairment of memory functions
    Reduction of sensory processes
    Impairment of multisynaptic neurotransmission
    Impairment of neuroendocrine functions

are listed in Table I. One of the most characteristic morphological changes in the human brain is a significant (10-20%) loss of brain weight believed to be due to a decrease in total brain protein and lipids. There is no loss of total brain water. Associated with the decrease in brain weight is a decreased brain volume leading to the shrunken and exaggerated convolutions with narrow gyri and deeper sulci. The volume of cerebrospinal fluid increases in relation to the change in ventricle volume which may slightly increase with normal aging but increases by 30% in dementia.

The weight changes are sometimes taken as evidence that the brain undergoes an age dependent loss of neurons. Other observations show that indeed there is a cell loss in cerebral cortex, cerebellum, locus coeruleus, and substantia nigra. There is no loss in many other areas, such as dentate nucleus, the nuclei of the many cranial nerves, and a number of brain stem nuclei.

In addition to cell loss, there is present neurofibrillary degeneration. In the normally aged, nearly 50% of the cases examined show neurofibrillary degeneration in some hippocampal neurons, and in 11% an occasional neuron affected in the neocortex.

An important structural change that is of interest is the loss of dendritic spines. Cortical pyramidal cells and cerebellar Purkinje cells in old animals and old humans have often been found to show greatly diminished numbers of dendritic spines per unit dendritic length. The human brain cells also show reduced dendritic arborization. The function of these spines seems to be a postsynaptic specialization to mediate synaptic input. This would then suggest that the loss of dendritic spines may alter the synaptic complement of the neurons and thus impair many synaptic functions including formation of memory traces.

Besides neuronal degeneration and loss of dendritic spines, there is frequent development of amyloid lesions, formation of senile (neuritic) plaques in neuronal perikarya, and intracytoplasmic development of neurofibrillary tangles. They are more characteristic of presenile and senile dementia and are less frequent in the brain of normal old people.

Among the neuropathological changes related to aging that we have found to be vulnerable to drug treatment is the accumulation of lipofuscin pigments. Because of its importance as a tool in drug development, a separate section is devoted to its discussion.

III. LIPOFUSCIN ACCUMULATION IN CNS

A. Lipofuscin in Mammalian Brain

Of the many histopathological changes of the brain, lipofuscin accumulation is one of the universally accepted cytoplasmic changes that are age related and are seen in the neurons, regardless of type or system and is universally present in all the mammals.

These pigments are most plentiful in nondividing cell types such as neurons and myocardium. Only small quantities have been demonstrated in liver, striated muscles, adrenal gland, and gonads. It has also been demonstrated that the amount of the pigment in human myocardium is proportional to age and it increases at a rate of approximately 0.6% of the total intracellular volume per decade (27). Its progressive increase with age has been studied in sympathetic ganglia and in the nuclei of central nervous system. Data from our experiments are shown in Figures 1 & 2 and were reviewed recently (18, 19). The neurons of the CNS of rodents exhibit a variable pattern of pigmentation in their cytoplasm. During the

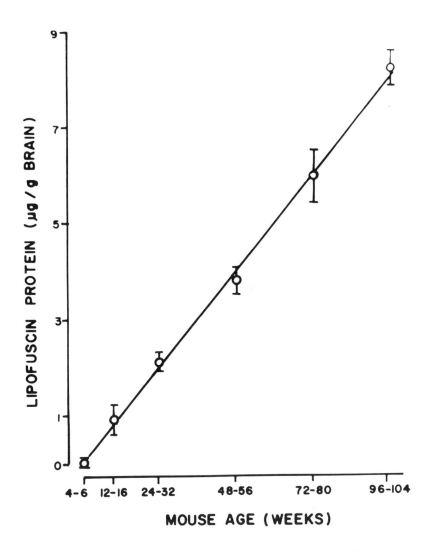

FIGURE 1 Lipofuscin content of brain in mice as function of age.

first two months it is hardly detectable. Subsequently it develops in diffuse fashion. In older animals, it surrounds the nucleus and forms clumps near the axon hillock or dendrites. The number of non-pigmented cells steadily decrease in number with age, from 100% in the newborn to 20% at 24 months in mice. Also, the rate of deposition differs from one brain area to another; the hippocampus

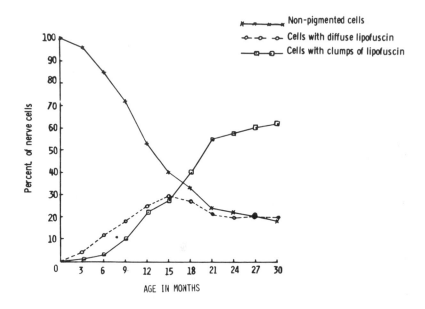

Non-pigmented cells

Cells with diffuse lipofuscin

Cells with clumps of lipofuscin

FIGURE 2   Lipofuscin distribution in pyramidal cells of cerebral cortex (layer III) in mice of different ages.

being the highest in concentration. It can be seen to increase with age in a somewhat linear fashion in mice (18), nonhuman primates (2), in guinea pigs (17, 29), dogs (28), pigs (28), and human (14, 22, 11). Studies in nonhuman primate (Macaca mulatta) has shown that lipofuscin pigment accumulation exhibits a regional variation which is highest in the medulla, and decreases in order, in hippocampus, midbrain, pons, neocortex, and the least in the cerebellum and hypothalmus (29). Similar studies with guinea pigs (29), rat (21) and mouse (21) have shown a high degree of hippocampal and medullary involvement. In humans, most histopathological changes occur maximally in cortical tissue, particularly in the cortex of the hippocampal complex (13). The regional occurrences of this pigment directly coincide with centers for cognitive learning and considerable work has demonstrated memory dysfunction as well as impairment of other behavioral and mental tasks in the aged (6, 7, 9, 12, 18).

The pigment is easily identified by histochemical characteristics and can be described as yellowish-brown granules or globules (light microscopy) and practically insoluble in fat solvents. The component materials are sudanophilic, PAS positive with a characteristic autofluorescence (yellow-green under UV light), seen within a limiting single membrane structures which are dispersed in neuronal cytoplasm. Approximately 56% of the dry weight of lipofuscin is dry material; possibly a polymeric lipid and phosopholid structure with amino acids, either bound to the lipids or as included protein. The electron microscopic studies have suggested the possible origin of the pigment in various cell-organelles (mitochondrial, Golgi complex, endoplasmic reticulum). Glees *et al.*, (8) presented some evidence of mitochondrial origin of neuronal lipofuscin; the majority of the electron microscopic studies, however, favor its lysosomal origin.

Lipofuscin pigments have been reported in excessive amounts in the neurons of subjects inflicted with various neuropathological conditions with shortened life span. An early formation of lipofuscin in abnormally high quantities has been reported in patients with Progeria and Warner's syndrome. Similar observations were made in a group of mutant mice who appeared to have a condition of premature aging. The animals usually die within 8 weeks of age, but lipofuscin pigment in their brain specimen is comparable to that in neurons of 12 month old mice. Excessive lipofuscin is also found in Batten-Vogt syndrome.

In addition to the natural process of aging, the lipofuscin accumulation in the central nervous system may be increased by other factors that cause prolonged insult or trauma to the cell. These factors include hypoxia, dietary vitamin E deficiency, and drugs such as acetanilid which produces cellular hypoxia or other toxic compounds such as tetraethylthiuram disulfide. Very recently dietary protein deficiency (4% and 8% protein calories) during gestation was shown to promote lipofuscin accumulation in the neonatal brain.

The lipofuscin accumulation due to the vitamin E deficient diet is used for experimental purposes because of the relative ease with which large numbers of animals can be affected. As is seen from data summarized in Table II, lipofuscin accumulation can be markedly enhanced in several brain areas by feeding the rats a vitamin E deficient diet. Once the accumulation levels reach a desired level, the normal diet can be restored without losing lipofuscin. In this way, the experimental animals can be used in repeated tests of learning and memory or used for various treatments to determine effects on lipofuscin related neurochemical dysfunctions. There is evidence that this type of induced pigment, although slightly different from natural pigment with respect to distribution of early and late types (15), can be consistently associated with a predictable course of accumulation and can be shown to cause aging-like deterioration of brain functions in normal animals (12, 18).

TABLE II

Enhancement of lipofuscin accumulation in the rat brain by vitamin E free diet.

	Lipofuscin Granules/10 Reticules Mean ± S.E.		
	Cortex*	Cerebellum**	Hippocampus***
Young	6 ± 5	5 ± 1.4	3 ± 1.7
Aged Control	45 ± 21	46 ± 9	51 ± 23
E-deficient Diet	73 ± 21	70 ± 11	145 ± 35

* Ventrolateral perietal cerebral cortex.
** Purkinje cells of granular layer.
*** Lateral and ventral pyramidal cells.
From Lal, H., Pogacar, S., Daly, P.R. and Puri, S.K.: Behavioral and neuropathological manifestations of nutritionally induced central nervous system aging in the rat. *Prog. Brain Res.* 40:129-142 (1973), with permission.

B. Lipofuscin in Neuroblastoma Cell Culture

Because of complexity of neuronal organization in whole animal and difficulties in obtaining neurosystems susceptible to relatively rapid study of aging, one must resort to *in vitro* models. Several preparations of nerve tissue have been described which may be used to study the process of aging in neuronal tissue. They include organ cultures, nerve tissue explants, and reaggregating the dispersed cell cultures. Most of these preparations, although useful for morphological and electrophysiological studies, are limited by being a coupled mixture of cell types. In addition, preparations obtained from mature and/or aged animals are less likely to yield functionally intact preparations since with age dissociation of neuronal tissue into single cells becomes difficult.

We found neuroblastoma cells in tissue culture to offer several advantages as a model system for neuronal aging. It is possible to obtain relatively large numbers of cells of a single type and ma-

Future Drugs against Senescence

nipulate their environment in which they are maintained. They can be prepared for drug treatment and analysis of effects without having to resort to traumatic isolation procedures. They can be maintained in a postmitotic nondividing state for long periods to induce occurrence of age-related changes.

Mouse neuroblastoma cells originally established in culture in 1969 have been studied for age-related changes. A characteristic feature of this cell type is that in culture the rapidly dividing tumor cells can be converted into nondividing cells with many properties similar to those of mature nerve cells. Various characteristics of these cells in culture have been recently reviewed by Schneider *et al.*, (24).

Mouse neuroblastoma cells in log growth, with generating times generally around 24 h, are round or slightly irregular shaped with diameters of approximately 25 to 40 μ. Usually 10-20% of the cells in log growth phase possess neurite-like processes.

Inhibition of cell division can be accomplished by a wide variety of manipulations which induce differentiation (16, 20). Once inhibited, these cells grow neurite-like processes which are morphologically similar to nerve axon in several ways. They frequently contain long microtubules, an axial bundle of filaments, and numerous microfilaments (10). The neurites also contain clusters of 400-600 Å diameter vesicles which are morphologically similar to synaptic vesicles.

The neuroblastoma cells which have formed neurites show increased activity of acetylcholinesterase, choline acetyltransferase, tyrosine hydroxylase, and dopamine-β-hydroxylase. These cells are capable of accumulating and metabolizing various neurotransmitters (1). Electrophysiological and biochemical studies have shown that neuroblastoma cells possess neurotransmitter and hormone receptors which are involved in electrical changes and alterations in levels of cyclic nucleolids.

Many receptor binding sites have been established to be located on neuroblastoma cell membranes. They include muscarine and nicotinic receptors, alpha adrenergic and dopaminergic receptors, and opioid or endorphin receptors.

We have investigated a number of agents to obtain populations of nondividing cells for the study of aging. One can successfully use low pH or the serum concentration of the medium, addition of papaverine, prostaglandin E, or other similar agents.

A number of age-related changes have been identified in neuroblastoma cells which are maintained in a nondividing state. They include formation of lipofuscin pigment, changes in lysosomal enzyme levels and acetylcholinesterase activity, growth of cell size and neurite-like processes, cell viability, and a characteristic latency for cell division upon reseeding. These changes were recently reviewed by Schneider *et al.*, (24). Lipofuscin accumulation can also be shown in other cell lines such as nondividing W1-38 human fibroblasts (4), glia cells (3), or in cultured dorsal root ganglion cells of the rat (26).

C. Functional Significance of Lipofuscin Accumulation

Although accumulation of lipofuscin during aging is well documented, its relationship with the functioning of nerve cells is unknown. To obtain reliable data in this respect it is necessary to study the neuronal functions before and after lipofuscin accumulation and establish that the deficit in the neuronal functions is restored after the removal of lipofuscin. Unfortunately a number of methodological difficulties do not permit successful studies of this type. In the absence of these studies, speculations based upon a variety of coincidental studies are offered. The studies in which Vitamin E deficient diet was used to enhance lipofuscin accumulation or those in which centrophenoxine was used to reduce neuronal lipofuscin suggest that there are many behavioral tasks related to memory and learning that deteriorate when lipofuscin levels are increased and the same tasks improve when lipofuscin levels are reduced. The learning paradigms which have been shown to be defected in conditions where higher accumulation of lipofuscin is found, are listed in Table 3.

TABLE III
Behavioral tasks which have been observed to show deficits with increasing lipofuscin in the mouse or rat brain.

Reversal learning of maze performance

Learning of conditional avoidance response

Recall of previously learned conditional avoidance responses

Delayed alternation of lever pressing responses

Recall of one trial aversive experience

Future Drugs against Senescence

It is difficult to state if the lipofuscin is a cause or effect of the age related brain dysfunctions. However, the results of morphological and biochemical studies indicate that the pigment is at least the wear and tear of the cellular constituents associated with aging, and the accumulation probably represents inability of the post-mitotic cells to dispose of the metabolic "garbage." Whether this "garbage" itself is harmful to the cells cannot be stated for sure. Lipofuscin may just represent the ashes after the fire rather than a causative factor. But, it is not unreasonable to expect that the presence of large amounts of "garbage" material which occupies a substantial part of the cell cytoplasm is detrimental to smooth functioning of the cells. Physical location of the lipofuscin at the origin of dendrites and nerve fibers is expected to at least retard the flow of the material from the cell body to the nerve endings.

D. Drug Effects on Lipofuscin Accumulation

(1) Guinea Pig

The effects of centrophenoxine on the lipofuscin pigment in the neurons in the brain of senile guinea pigs were studied using histological and histochemical methods. Mostly older animals (3-4 years) were used in this study. They were treated with centrophenoxine (80 mg/kg of body weight) by intraperitoneal injection daily for 4-16 weeks. The pigments accumulated steadily in the neurons of control animals with the increase of age, and a notable diminution of lipofuscin pigments was observed in most parts of the CNS in the treated animals. The degree of the effect of the drug was largely dependent on the duration of the treatment and a marked reduction was observed after 12 weeks or more. The effects of the drug on the activities of succinate, lactate, and glucose-6-phosphate dehydrogenases, cytochrome oxidase, acid phosphatase, and simple esterase were also studied in these animals. There was an appreciable reduction of the activity of succinate and lactate dehydrogenases, simple esterase, and acid phosphatase and this effect was most marked in the area of deposition of the pigment. The activity of glucose-6-phosphate dehydrogenase, on the other hand, was appreciably increased, and this was evident throughout the cytoplasm of the neurons. It was, therefore, suggested that the drug may help to reduce lipofuscin pigment by a possible diversion of the glucose metabolism from Krebs cycle to pentose shunt and also by depression of lysosomal activity. A parallel histochemical study on the enzymatic activities of the motor neurons of the spinal cord during regeneration following axonal injury was also carried out in young and old guinea pigs. It was rather interesting to note that the regenerating neurons also metabolized glucose via pentose cycle, in addition to or bypassing tricarboxylic acid and glycolytic pathways during recovery from injury.

(2) Mice

As mice are the most widely used experimental animals, they were employed in the aging studies. Recently, one month old mice were treated with centrophenoxine by intraperitoneal injection (80 mg/kg of body weight) up to 11 months and a similar number of the same without treatment were used as controls. Five mice were sacrificed from both groups after 2, 5, 8, and 11 months of treatment. The study indicated that the drug did not stop lipofuscin formation even when the treatment was started before the onset of pigmentogenesis. On the other hand, there was a consistent decrease in the pigment in the neurons of cerebral cortex and hippocampus in the treated animals compared to the age-matched controls. The degree of reduction was largely dependent on the duration of the treatment and a significant diminution was noted after treatment for 5 months or more. These data are illustrated in Figure 3.

In the past years, the effects of centrophenoxine on already accumulated lipofuscin was studied in cerebral cortex and hippocampus. Eleven to twelve-month-old female mice were treated with centrophenoxine (80 mg/kg of body weight) for three months and their learning and memory were tested in a T-maze. There was a substantial reduction of lipofuscin pigment in the cerebral cortex and hippocampus demonstrated by its characteristic autofluorescence, histochemical, and ultrastructural properties. Reduction in brain lipofuscin by chronic treatment with centrophenoxine is illustrated in Figure 3. A significant reduction is consistently observed after three months of treatment compared to the control group of the same age, both in the neurons of the cerebral cortex and the hippocampus as illustrated in Figure 3. The electron microscopic studies showed that the centrophenoxine treatment causes lipofuscin pigments to be fragmented so that progressive fragmentation causes formation of microglobules which disappear either by enzymatic digestion or leakage. The process of fragmentation is illustrated in Figure 4.

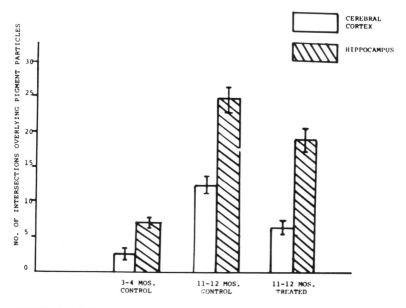

FIGURE 3   Effect of centrophenoxine on brain lipofuscin content.

(3) Neuroblastoma Cells in Culture

C1300 mouse neuroblastoma cells in culture were used to study cytoplasmic lipofuscin pigment accumulation and the ability of centrophenoxine to alter its formation. The pigment was detected by its autofluorescence and histochemical staining for acid Schiff procedure. The percentage of the cells with pigment increased from 20% at 5 days to 50% by day 25 of culture. Pigment formation was enhanced by treatment for 9 days with either 1.1×10^{-5}M papaverine or 5.6×10^{-5}M prostaglandin E_1. Pigment formation in papaverine treated cells was markedly reduced by treatment for 9 days with either 1.0×10^{-4}M or 3.4×10^{-4}M centrophenoxine added daily to the culture media. These data are illustrated in Table 4. The drug in those concentrations did not decrease cell viability, increase cell sloughing, or significantly alter cell growth over the time period of these studies (23).

An electron microscopic study was carried out on the effects of centrophenoxine on the lipofuscin pigment in uncloned (T59) and cloned (NBA2) mouse C1300 neuroblastoma cells in culture. Cells were grown in monolayer in T75 falcon plastic flasks containing 10 ml of Ham's chemically defined synthetic medium (FIBCO Ham's F-12). Cells were maintained at 36°C in humidified air containing

63

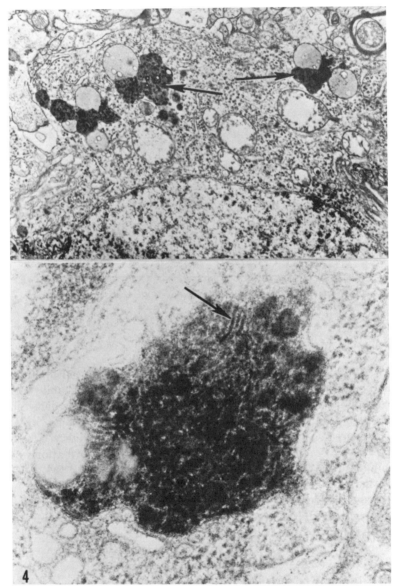

FIGURE 4   Electron microscopic characterization of lipofuscin nerve cells.

5% CO_2 and were routinely subcultured every four or five days to maintain logarithmic growth. Cells were harvested for transfer for analysis by exposure for 6 min at 36°C to 2 ml of 0.25% Viokase in phosphate-buffered saline. Cell counts were made with a Model

Future Drugs against Senescence

TABLE IV
Effectiveness of centrophenoxine in reducing lipofuscin
in the neuroblastoma cell in tissue culture.

Drug	Concentration	% Cells with Lipofuscin
None	—	33 ± 2
Papaverine	1.1×10^{-5}M	51 ± 4
Papaverine + Centrophenoxine	30 mg/ml	45 ± 3
Papaverine + Centrophenoxine	100 mg/ml	23 ± 2

From Nandy, K. and Schneider, H.: Lipofuscin pigment formation in neuroblastoma cells in culture. Neurobiol. Aging 8:245-265 (1976), with permission.

D-2 Coulter automatic blood cell counter. Centrophenoxine was added to culture daily for three weeks beginning three days after initial seeding; final concentration of the drug was either 10^{-4} or 3.4×10^{-4}M.

Cells were prepared for electron microscopic examination by the following procedure: Medium was removed from the cells and replaced by 10 ml of serum-free media which was left on the cells for 60 min at 37°C. After removing the serum-free media, the cells were harvested by gentle scraping with a rubber policeman, removed with 2 ml of serum-free media, and centrifuged for 10 min at 1,000 rpm. The resulting pellet was fixed in Karnovsky's paraformaldehyde-gluteraldehyde mixture, postfixed in phosphate-buffered 1% osmium tetroxide, dehydrated in a graded series of alcohols, and embedded in a meraglass-cardolite mixture. Ultrathin sections were cut with an LKB-Ultratome III ultramicrotome and were mounted on espper grids and stained with uranyl acetate and lead citrate. Microscopy was carried out with an RCA EMU-3D electron microscope. Electron dense materials similar to lipofuscin granules in size, morphology, and distribution were present in only small quantities in T59 neuroblastoma cells three days after seeding. Virus particles were evident and mitochondrial structure was normal. However, pigment was quite noticeable in cultures by day 10 as tightly packed electron-dense bodies located in the cytoplasm, along with lipid droplets, swollen mitochondria, and the virus particles. Although the percent of the cells which contain pigment is only slightly higher after 20 days in culture than after 10 days (16), each cell actually contains more highly developed pigment formations. The electron-dense whorls of tightly packed membrane material mainly composed the pigment granules.

This study indicated that the addition of centrophenoxine (3.4 × 10^{-4}M) for nine days can prevent the increase in pigment. The results are even more marked when both papaverine, a phosphodiesterase inhibitor (10^{-5}M), and centrophenoxine were added for nine days. There are fewer pigment granules and the appearance of the pigment is similar to that observed for untreated cells. When neuroblastoma cells are treated with papaverine and centrophenoxine for 19 days, there is a further reduction of pigment and an increase in the rough endoplasmic reticulum. This study further confirms the light microscopic observation on the effects of centrophenoxine on lipofuscin in neuroblastoma cells using electron-microscopic methods (18).

IV. BRAIN NEUROTRANSMITTER CHANGES IN AGING BRAIN

A. Neurotransmitters and Brain Functions

The CNS is organized to perform its functions through neuronal intercommunications that are accomplished at billions of synapses. At a synapse, a neurotransmitter is released from the presynaptic sites as a result of presynaptic neuronal activity. This transmitter then diffuses in the synaptic gap to the sites where specific receptors for this neurotransmitter are located. The transmitter is attracted by the receptors to which it binds. The receptors are structurally specialized spots on the nerve membrane which show high binding affinity for specific neurotransmitters. These receptors contain a transduction mechanism that allows neurotransmitter binding with the receptor to translate itself into physicochemical sequelae that lead ultimately to the deserved response. The nature of the transducing mechanisms remains a "black box"; however, a few efforts to penetrate this box ought to be mentioned.

Cyclic neucleotides have been proposed to act as "second messengers" in a number of catecholamine (CA) controlled synaptic actions in the CNS. In order to accomplish this, specific and synapse specific nucleotides (cyclic AMP and cyclic GMP) are produced by the action of neurotransmitters on a class of enzymes called nucleotide cyclases.

Over the past 25 years, progressive analysis of the synthesis,

storage, release, conservation, and catabolism of brain neurotransmitters has pointed out the role of these neurotransmitters in
many brain functions, mental disease states, and bases for pharmacological intervention in a variety of situations. However, research on the changes in the neurotransmitter functions that occur
in the senescence-related brain dysfunctions is in its infancy as a
scientific discipline.

Among the neurotransmitters that have been considered important in brain functioning are included acetylcholine, catecholamines, serotonin, and gamma-aminobutyric acid (GABA).

B. Cholinergic System

Acetylcholine (ACh) is an established neurotransmitter substance
of the cholinergic system. ACh is synthesized from acetic acid and
choline, a reaction catalysed by the enzyme choline acetyltransferase (CAT). ACh is present in the cytoplasm as well as in the
storage granules of the nerve ending. It is released into the synaptic
cleft where it acts on ACh specific receptors to produce "second
messenger" substance and is subsequently hydrolyzed by the enzyme acetylcholinesterase. The degradation products acetic acid
and choline are recycled for ACh synthesis.

Among the functions in which the cholinergic system is implicated
are included learning, memory, neuroendocrine functioning, and
motor coordination. The brain levels of ACh in aged animals do not
differ from those of adult animals. However, the brain levels of
ACh in old animals are significantly reduced by administration of
d-amphetamine given in a dose that is ineffective in the adult animal (5). This observation suggests that ACh turnover in the brains
of old animals may be differentially sensitive to drugs that act
through catecholaminergic mechanisms.

Most investigators agree that the activity of both ACh and CAT
are reduced in some brain areas of senescent mice and rats, and
there may be a change also in the turnover rate of brain acetylcholine. However, most of the experiments in this area are only
preliminary and concrete information on acetylcholine turnover
may not be available until more accurate methods of the turnover
measurements become available.

An aspect of cholinergic functions that is intimately related to the
drug action is the observation that there is change in the responsivity of the cholinergic systems to stimulation in the aged animal.
The threshold dose of ACh given into the cerebral ventricles to pro-

Psychotropic Drug Research

duce EEG, cardiovascular and respiratory changes is much smaller in the aged animals. The most pronounced alteration in ACh response occurs in the sensorimotor cortex, hippocampus, and amygdala. Our preliminary observations using the *in vivo* procedures of employing selected drugs to determine cholinergic responsivity in the whole animal show that the aged animals are far more sensitive to the cholinomimetic drugs than their adult counterpart. There is hyperresponsivity to the cholinergic agonist (see Table V) and decreased sensitivity to the pharmacological effects of cholinergic antagonists (see Table VI). These observations, although only preliminary, suggest that there may be important changes in the receptor mechanisms of the cholinergic systems. If it is so confirmed by future research, various pharmacological approaches should be considered to both prevent and treat this neurotransmitter dysfunction. Also, one may exercise a caution in using the cholinergic drugs in the aged population as their responses may be unpredictable.

TABLE V
Changes in sensitivity to oxotremorine, the effects on locomotor activity in aged mice.

Age (months)	N	% Inhibition of Locomotor Activity Mean ± S.E.
3-5	10	26 ± 7
14-18	10	83 ± 3

TABLE VI
Changes in sensitivity to the effects of dexetimide in locomotor activity in aged mice.

Age (months)	N	% Stimulation of Locomotor Activity Mean ± S.E.
3-5	15	78 ± 5
14-18	15	19 ± 3

C. Catecholaminergic Systems

The CNS contains three types of catecholamines: dopamine (DA), norepinephrine (NE), and epinephrine. Among them DA neuron systems are more complex in their anatomy, more diverse in localization and functions, and more numerous, both in terms of definable systems and in number of neurons, than the other catecholamine systems. Therefore, we are paying more attention to the study of DA systems.

DA neuron systems are principally located in the upper mesencephalon and diencephalon. They vary anatomically from systems of neurons without axons (retina, olfactory bulb) and with very restricted projections, to systems with extensive axonal arborizations. In contrast to NE systems, the DA systems appear to be "local" systems with highly specified and topographically organized projections. The important DA systems are illustrated in Table VII.

In aged subjects, the enzyme tyrosine hydroxylase, which is critical in the synthesis of catecholamines, is found deficient in activity suggesting that catecholamine synthesis is reduced. This decrease in catecholamine synthesis is found in many areas of the brain. The synthesis decrease is not related to any deficit in the availability or uptake of catecholamine precursors.

In addition, there is a marked decrease in the levels of dopamine in the striatum without such change in the levels of NE in this area of the brain. These findings suggest that either the synthetic apparatus of neurons is damaged or that a significant number of neurons containing this apparatus have degenerated in the senescent subjects. Upon careful examination both deficits are found to occur. There is a marked decline in the synthetic enzymes as well as significant decreases in the DA cell population in the aged subjects. These findings have been reported to be present both in the senescent animal, as well as in the elderly human subjects.

In order to study the neurotransmitter release in the aged animal, we employ amphetamine, a drug which produces its stimulant action through release of dopamine. We found that the aged mice were markedly less responsive to the locomotor stimulating effects of amphetamine (Table VIII). Lack of anorexic and anti-insomniac effects of amphetamine-like drugs have been noticed in the elderly patients. Recently, reduced toxicity of phenylephrine was reported in the aged mice.

Besides our indirect evidence of deficits in release mechanism, it was found that the receptor sites also diminish in the aged animals. DA receptors can now be determined both *in vitro* and *in vivo* by the procedures developed in the last five years. Availability of highly specific receptor ligands have greatly contributed to these advances.

In recent years new methods have been developed to characterize receptor population for various neurotransmitters in discrete brain

TABLE VII

Dopamine neuron systems in the mammalian brain.

System	Nucleus of Origin	Site(s) of Termination
Meso-telencephalic Nigrostriatal	Substantia nigra, pars compacta; ventral tegmental area	Neostriatum (caudate putamen) globus pallidus
Mesocortical	Ventral tegmental area; substantia nigra, pars compacta	Iscortex (mesial frontal, anterior cingulate, entorhinal, perirhinal) Allocortex (olfactory bulb, anterior olfactory nucleus, olfactory tubercle, piriform cortex, septal area, nucleus accumbens, amygdaloid complex)
Tubero-hypophysial	Arcuate and periventricular hypothalamic nuclei	Neuro-intermediate lobe of pituitary, median eminence
Incerto-hypothalamic	Zona incerta, posterior hypothalamus	Dorsal hypothalamic area, septum
Periventricular	Medulla in area of dorsal motor vagus, nucleus tractus solitarius, periaqueductal and periventricular gray	Periventricular and peri-aqueductal gray, tegmentum, tectum, thalamus, hypothalamus
Olfactory bulb	Periglomerular cells	Glomeruli (mitral cells)
Retinal	Interplexiform cells of retina	Inner and outer plexiform layers of retina

Future Drugs against Senescence

Differential stimulation of locomotor activity by
amphetamine in mice of different ages.

Age (months)	N	% Stimulation of Locomotor Activity Mean ± S.E.
3-5	10	62 ± 11
14-17	30	28 ± 7
25-30	10	0

areas. Briefly speaking, the homogenates of different brain areas
are incubated with a suitable receptor ligand which is previously
made radioactive in order to trace minute quantities that are bound
to the receptors. In the study on senescence the brain dopamine
receptors have been labelled with H^3-haloperidol or H^3-spiroperidol.
Sufficient quantities of the ligand are used to reach binding equilibrium, following which the radioactive ligand bound to the receptor membrane is separated from the free and nonspecifically bound
quantities for quantitative determination. The specifically bound
ligand to the receptor is distinguished from nonspecific binding by
including suitably selected nonradioactive drugs in the incubation.
The stereospecifically active form of these drugs displaces only
specifically bound ligand while the biologically nonactive stereois-
omer of the drug displaces the ligand only from the nonspecific
binding sites. This procedure narrows down most of the bindings to
specific receptor sites.

In the study of the aged animals including primates, both H^3-
haloperidol and H^3-spiroperidol as well as two stereoisomers of butaclamol have been employed. In all cases it was found that there
was an appreciable decrease in the number of receptor binding sites
in the brain samples obtained from the aged animals. A decrease in
the dopamine receptor binding sites is particularly significant in
caudate-putamen, frontal cortex, and various areas of anterior limbic cortex. A further analysis of these data shows that changes in
binding characteristics are exclusively due to a reduction in the
number of the binding sites. The affinity of the remaining receptors to the dopamine antagonists is not altered (Mackman, personal communication).

The observation that there is a significant decrease in the dopaminergic neuron functioning in the aged has many implications.

Psychotropic Drug Research

First of all, the high vulnerability of dopaminergic neurons in the aged requires preventive measures to protect these neurons from further damage. New drugs may be synthesized to stimulate synthesis and regeneration of various components. Regeneration of neuronal spines, dendrites, and the receptor population is not beyond the currently known capabilities of the pharmacological tools. Many prototype pharmacological procedures are known in this field.

Whereas the deficient dopaminergic systems in the aged may be a cause of concern in most cases, it is suggested that it may be helpful for the schizophrenics. Reduction in dopaminergic activity is often employed as a treatment modality in the schizophrenics. Most neuroleptics are believed to work through this mechanism. However, if the current hypotheses of schizophrenia are true, the aging process is expected to produce spontaneous remission of many of the symptoms related to this disease.

V. CONCLUSION

Neuropathological changes associated with senescence include structural as well as neurochemical alterations. Lipofuscin accumulation may serve as an easily measurable index of many complex changes. Receptor binding, assays, changes in sensitivity to selected drugs, and measurement of the cyclase may serve as measures of critical neurochemical changes. For drug development research neuroblastoma cells in tissue culture may serve as an easy target to determine drug effects on lipofuscin accumulation. Mice and rats given a vitamin E deficient diet may serve as a whole animal model to screen drugs with anti-senility functions. Other methods of developing animal models of senility are being developed through immunological manipulations but they are not yet available for drug development research. Besides a search for drugs to reverse the neuropathological process, other drugs which allow neurotransmitter functions may also be useful. Many drugs are currently being employed to reverse the process of neurotransmitter receptor degeneration.

REFERENCES

1. Breakefield, X.O.: Neurotransmitter metabolism in murine neuroblastoma cells. *Life Sci.* 18:267-278, 1976.
2. Brizzee, K.R., Harkin, J.C., Ordy, S.M. and Kaack, B.: Accumulation and distribution of lipofuscin, amyloid and senile plaques in the aging

nervous system. In H. Brody, D. Harman and J.M. Ordy (Eds.), *Aging.* Volume I, Raven Press, New York, 1975, pp. 39-78.

3. Brunk, U., Ericsson, J.L.E., Ponter, J. and Westermark, B.: Residual bodies and "aging" in cultured human glial cells. *Exp. Cell Res.* 79:1-14, 1973.

4. Deamer, D.W., Gonzales, J.: Autofluorescent structures in cultured WI-38 cells. *Arch. Biochem. Biophys.* 165:421-426, 1964.

5. Domino, E.F., Dren, A.T. and Glardina, W.J.: Biochemical and neurotransmitter changes in the aging brain. In M.A. Lipton, A. DiMascio and K.F. Killam (Eds.), *Psychopharmacology: A Generation of Progress,* Raven Press, New York, 1978, pp. 1507-1515.

6. Doty, B.: Age and avoidance conditioning in rats. *J. Geront.* 21:287-290, 1966.

7. Dye, C.J.: Effect of interruption of initial learning upon retention in young, mature and old rats. *J. Geront.* 24:12-17, 1969.

8. Glees, P., Hasan, M., and Tischner, K.: The cytological distribution of osmiophilic bodies in the normal and degenerating lateral geniculate nucleus of the monkey. An electron microscopic study. *Acta Neuropath.* 8:285-291, 1967.

9. Gordon, P., Tobin, S.S., Doty, B. and Nash, M.: Drugs effect on behavior in aged animals and man: Diphenylhydantoin and procainamide. *J. Geront.* 23:434-444, 1973.

10. Hinkley, R.E. and Telser, A.G.: The effects of halothane on cultured mouse neuroblastoma cells. I. Inhibition of morphological differentiation. *J. Cell. Biol.* 63:531-540, 1974.

11. Issidorides, M. and Shanklin, W.M.: Histochemical reaction of cellular inclusion in the human neuron. *J. Anat.* (London) 95:151-159, 1961.

12. Lal, H., Pogacar, S., Daly, P.R. and Puri, S.K.: Behavioral and neuropathological manifestations of nutritionally induced central nervous system aging in the rat. *Prog. Brain Res.* 40:129-142, 1973.

13. Malamud, N.: Neuropathology of organic brain syndrome associated with aging. In C.M. Gaity (Ed.), *Aging and the Brain,* Plenum Press, New York, 1972.

14. Mann, D.M.A. and Yates, P.O.: Lipoprotein pigments—their relationship to aging in the human nervous system. I. The lipofuscin content of nerve cells. *Brain* 97:481-488, 1974.

15. Nandy, K.: Properties of neuronal lipofuscin in mice. *Acta Neuropathol.* 19:25-32, 1971.

16. Nandy, K. and Schneider, H.: Lipofuscin pigment formation in neuroblastoma cells in culture. In R. Terry and S. Gershin (Eds.), *Neurobiololgy of Aging,* Raven Press, New York, 1976, pp. 245-264.

17. Nandy, K.: Further studies on the effects of centrophenoxine on the lipofuscin pigment in the neurons of senile guinea pigs. *J. Geront.* 23:82-92, 1968.

18. Nandy, K. and Lal, H.: Neuronal lipofuscin and learning deficits in aging mammals. *Prog. Neuropsychopharm,* 1978.

19. Nandy, K.: Morphological changes in the aging brain, In K. Nandy (Ed.), *Senile Dementia: A Biomedical Approach,* Elsevier/North Holland, New York 1978, pp. 19-32.
20. Prasad, K.N.: Differentiation of neuroblastoma cells in culture. *Biol. Rev.* 50:129-165, 1975.
21. Reichel, W., Hollander, J., Clark, J. and Strehler, B.L.: Lipofuscin pigment accumulation as a function of age and distribution in rodent brain. *J. Geront.* 23:71-78, 1968.
22. Samorajski, T., Ordy, J.M. and Pady-Peimer, P.: Lipofuscin pigment accumulation in the nervous system of aging mice. *Anat. Rec.* 16:555-562, 1968.
23. Schneider, H. and Nandy, K.: Effects of centrophenoxine on lipofuscin formation in neuroblastoma cells in culture. *J. Geront.* 32:132-139, 1977.
24. Schneider, H., Rehnberg, S.G. and Beer, M.P.: Aging of neurons in culture. In K. Nandy and I. Sherwin (Eds.), *The Aging Brain and Senile Dementia,* Plenum Press, New York, 1977b, pp. 157-178.
25. Siegel, J.S.: Some demographic aspects of aging in the United States. In A.M. Ostefeld and D.C. Gibson (Eds.), *Epidemiology of Aging,* U.S. Government Printing Office, Washington, 1975, pp. 17-82.
26. Spoerri, P.E. and Glees, P.: Neuronal aging in cultures: An electromicroscopic study. *Exp. Geront.* 8:259-263, 1973.
27. Strehler, B.L., Mark, D.D., Mildman, A.S. and Gee, M.V.: Rate and magnitude of age pigment accumulation in the human myocardium. *J. Geront.* 14:430-439, 1959.
28. Whiteford, R. and Getty, R.: Distribution of lipofuscin in canine and porcine brain as related to aging. *J. Geront.* 21:31-44, 1966.
29. Wilcox, H.H.: Structural changes in the nervous sytem related to the process of aging. In Birren, Imus and Windle (Eds.), *The Process of Aging in the Nervous System.* Charles C Thomas, Springfield, 1959, Chap. 2, pp. 16-39.

4

Psychopharmacology in Geropsychiatry: Present and Future

THOMAS A. BAN, M.D.

I. EPIDEMIOLOGICAL DATA

As a result of the increase in average life expectancy at birth, of the three billion people living today, approximately 200 million are aged. There are approximately 22 million persons 65 years old and older (or approximately 30 million persons 60 years and older) in the United States, and it is estimated that by the year 2025 their total number will rise to over 42 million. Even with conservative estimates the number of old people will be almost doubled within the next 50 years (65, 99).

There is a high incidence of psychiatric morbidity in the aged. During the first half of the century a three-to fourfold increase in the number of persons over 65 years was associated with a ninefold increase in the number of first admissions from this age group to mental hospitals in the United States. In spite of the sharp reduction in admission rates to mental hospitals for all age ranges during the period from 1958 to 1968, first admission rates in 1965 were about 70 per 100,000 for the age group under 65, 100 per 100,000 for the age group 65 to 74, and as high as 200 per 100,000 for the age group 75 to 84 (80, 81, 92).

The rapid increase in individuals of 65 years or older in the general population has directed attention to gerontology, the scientific study of the aging process, and geriatrics, the medical specialty concerned with the study, prevention, and treatment of pathological conditions in the aged. Gerontology deals with primary aging, or senescence, which is a biological process rooted in heredity, and geriatrics deals with secondary aging, or senility, i.e., defects and disabilities resulting from trauma, including disease. The high

Presented at the Hoechst-Roussel Pharmaceuticals Inc. Research Seminar "New Frontiers in Psychotropic Drug Research," Hershey, Pennsylvania, October 18, 1978.

incidence of psychiatric morbidity in old people has created a need for the development of geropsychiatry, or psychogeriatrics, specially concerned with psychiatric disorders in the aged (7, 18).

While psychopathological symptoms and syndromes are similar in the young and the old, certain psychopathological manifestations, such as delirium, dysmnesia, and dementia are more common, and others, such as depression, anxiety, and delusions are modified in patients above 65 years old. Similarly, certain mental disorders such as arteriosclerotic or multi-infarct dementia, Alzheimer's disease, and senile psychosis are more common, and others, such as neurosis, manic-depressive illness, and schizophrenia are modified in this age group. Furthermore, interference with everyday functioning, including sleep and sexual behaviors, are rather frequent in aged subjects and geropsychiatric patients.

II. PREVENTIVE CONSIDERATIONS

In spite of the fourfold increase in average life expectancy at birth, the individual life span has remained unchanged throughout recorded history, and the individual "biological clock" begins to run out at about 85 to 100 years of age, even under the best possible environmental conditions, The reason for this is that increase in life expectancy to date has been exclusively due to "disease control," i.e., successful medical treatment of illness which in the past caused untimely death, and only in the light of some recent research contributions has extension of individual life span, through "rate control", become a distinct future possibility. Prerequisites of "rate control" are discoveries about the nature of the intrinsic biological process which regulates aging, and the slowing of the "biological clock" that is presumably operating (37, 59, 86, 99).

It is difficult to predict, however, which of the various theories of aging will be sufficiently substantiated by evidence to warrant the formulation of testable clinical pharmacological hypotheses of rate control. In the meantime, the fact remains that extension of life span into a period of the human life cycle where .physical and psychological changes which may seriously interfere with everyday functioning prevail, may not mean a true prolongation of life, but only a postponement of death.

III. EVERYDAY FUNCTIONING

Inverse sleep rhythm, with restlessness at night and sleepiness or drowsiness during the day, is one of the most common complaints in the aged. Appetite may be interfered with and sexual functioning is decreased.

A. Nighttime Behavior

Sleep requirements and patterns are considerably changed in the aged; elderly people require a longer period to fall asleep, sleep lighter, and experience more frequent awakenings. Awakenings increase from around two per night in the thirties, to as many as seven or eight per night in the eighties; duration of REM periods become more equalized with advancing age, and the deepest stages (III or IV) of sleep gradually diminish. Nevertheless, only in the ninth decade is there a significant reduction in total sleep time. In variance with the traditional view, that the elderly require less sleep, there is increasing evidence that as patients grow older sleep becomes more important to them (18, 22, 41, 95, 129, 135).

In view of these changes, an ideal hypnotic for the aged should provide for both rapid induction and long duration of sleep; should be free from paradoxical disinhibiting and delayed hypnotic effects; should not interfere with cortical brain metabolism to the extent that it produces a disturbance of consciousness; should increase stage IV sleep; and should decrease REM sleep which is often associated with frightening dreams and is possibly responsible for some of the cardiovascular or cerebrovascular accidents (85).

Among the various hypnotic preparations, barbiturates are contraindicated in geriatric patients because of the paradoxical reactions they may cause. While barbiturates in general decrease cerebral metabolism and thereby tend to increase agitation and confusion, Stotsky, Cole, and Tang (123) report that one of the slower acting barbiturates, sodium butabarbital, is both safe and effective in moderate doses for elderly patients with sleep disorders that are refractory to other hypnotics. Among the non-barbiturate hypnotics, chloral hydrate and paraldehyde have been used most frequently. During the 1960s they were replaced by chloral betaine, glutethimide, methyprylon, ethchlorvynol, methylparafynol, ethinamate, and methaqualone. Nevertheless, the fact remains that none of these drugs offer meaningful advantages over the barbiturates. In a recent report temazepam, a benzodiazepine hypnotic, was found to be a suitable sleep-inducer in geriatric patients. Nevertheless, Hollister (63) maintains that the benzodiazepines, flurazepam (15 mg to 30 mg) and triazolam (0.25 mg to 0.50 mg), are closest to meeting the characteristics of an ideal hypnotic (95, 97, 109).

Psychotropic Drug Research

While clinical trials with benzodiazepine hypnotics are still in progress, research efforts have been directed to explore the hypnotic properties of L-tryptophan, the precursor of tryptamine and serotonin, (a naturally occurring substance) and gamma-hydroxybutyrate, a normal metabolite found in the brain. Effectiveness and advantages of these substances in the treatment of insomnia in the aged remains to be seen (58, 63, 98).

B. Daytime Behavior

After a sleepless and restless night, sleepiness and drowsiness are frequently seen in the aged during the day. It was probably for this reason that the use of stimulant drugs has enjoyed a certain popularity. They have also been employed on the basis of the assumption that the greater fatigability, the general motor retardation, and decrease of drive and energy, all of which are characteristic of the waning powers of old age, would be specifically counteracted by central nervous system (CNS) stimulant drugs.

Among the various CNS stimulants, pentylenetetrazol is the most thoroughly studied. It has been evaluated in about 50 published clinical trials with geriatric patients. But of 16 controlled and comparative studies, only five produced clearly favorable clinical results. Although considerably less extensively studied, results of clinical trials with pipradrol (5 mg/day) are more favorable than with pentylenetetrazol. In all six clinical trials reviewed, five uncontrolled and one controlled, pipradrol produced beneficial effects. Results of clinical trials with methylphenidate are also more favorable than with pentylenetetrazol. Of the seven clinical trials reviewed methylphenidate (5 to 30 mg/day) produced beneficial effects in five. Nevertheless, in the one, 12-week comparative clinical study reviewed, no favorable therapeutic findings were seen (87, 108).

Numerous other known CNS stimulant drugs have been tried in geriatric patients. Among them, fencamfamin is a camphor derivative with alerting properties that has acquired some popularity in Europe. Magnesium pemoline was originally introduced with the hope that it would facilitate memory functions through an increase in the synthesis of ribonucleic acid. These expectations were not fulfilled. The modest benefits attributed to pemoline (37.5 to 150 mg/day) are now believed to be due to its mild stimulating effect. In this respect, pemoline may be somewhat more selective than other presently available CNS stimulant drugs (3, 64, 89).

There is no consensus about the use of CNS stimulants in geropsychiatric practice. On the basis of his clinical experience Lehmann (86) maintains that CNS stimulants are indicated for those geriatric patients who benefit if their vigilance, drive, and motivation is increased and their excessive fatigue diminished. However, if patients are excited, anxious, delusional, or hallucinated, those stimulants which lack adrenergic activity, such as caffeine, pemoline, and pentylenetetrazol should be given preference; while those with adrenergic activity such as amphetamine, fencamfamin, methylphenidate, and pipradrol should be used with caution. On the other hand, Hollister (64) argues that the increased cardiac work, irritability, decreased appetite, and possible aggravation of psychotic manifestations outweigh the questionable benefits of these drugs. Similarly, Prien (108) considers CNS stimulants of no apparent value in the treatment of the aged.

C. Sexual Behavior

It has been observed that conditional cues may fail to elicit conditional responses in the aged. Accordingly, smelling of food yields to little or no salivary secretion, and sexual fantasies alone only rarely result in full penile erection. In the aging male, even with persistent manual stimulation, it requires a longer period of time to achieve an erection; ejaculation is considerably delayed and is usually not accompanied by nipple erection. Similarly, in aging females, vaginal lubrication is delayed and decreased and painful contractions of the uterus may accompany orgasm. In both sexes there is a reduction of frequency in sexual needs. This may be overcome by the administration of androgens, paradoxically more reliably in females than in males. For some time estrogen has been successfully used to improve vaginal lubrication and stop painful uterine contractions; and recently there have been some indications that both L-Dopa (a dopamine precursor) and bromocriptine (a dopamine agonist) have a facilitating effect on erection. Furthermore, the possibility was raised that mesterolone, a synthetic androgen preparation, may not only lower erectile threshold, but also facilitates spermatogenesis and ejaculation (12, 18, 91, 105, 117).

In spite of all the promising leads to improve everyday functioning the fact remains that we have still problems in securing restful sleep and active days in the aged.

IV. GENERAL PSYCHOPATHOLOGY

A. Dysmnesia

Dysmnesia is the most frequent psychopathological manifestation in geropsychiatric patients. The memory disturbance may affect all three elementary memory functions, i.e., learning, or acquisition (formation of durable traces), retention, or preserving the material learned (consolidation of durable traces), and recall, or release of relevant material and its use in new situations. Impairment of recent memory, with well preserved remote and immediate memory functions is the most frequently encountered memory disorder in geropsychiatric patients. In view of this, the identification whether the memory disturbance includes immediate, recent and/or remote events is of the utmost diagnostic significance (5, 92).

A rare but characteristic psychopathological syndrome of old age is presbyophrenia, a condition in which memory impairment is seen .in seemingly well preserved geriatric patients. From a psychopathological point of view, however, most important is that seriously impaired (virtually absent) acquisition is associated with partially impaired retention for events occurring in the immediate and not too distant past in presbyophrenic patients (102).

In contrast to presbyophrenia, frequently occurring, but not characteristic acquisition disturbances of old age, are the amnesias. The memory gap may be confined to content (systematized) or more often to time (localized). On the basis of their completeness, localized amnesias are subdivided into total or partial; on the basis of their relationship to the disturbed state of consciousness into congrade, retrograde, and anterograde; and on the basis of their developmental course into transitory and retarded amnesias.

Other memory disturbances of old age include impaired retention, manifest in general (overall), or specific (lacunar) forgetfulness, seen in senile dementia and in arteriosclerotic dementia respectively, and disturbance of recall. Hypermnesia (excessive recall of details) for childhood events, may be simultaneously present with hypomnesia (decreased recall of details) for recent experiences, and infrequently with paramnesia (falsification of memory) and/or cryptamnesia. Some consider confabulations (the filling in of memory gaps by events which may or may not have occurred), a commonly seen psychopathological symptom in geropsychiatric patients, a distinct group of retroactive hallucinations. Nevertheless, while the content of retroactive hallucinations, a qualitative disturbance of recall, remains the same, the content of confabulations changes continuously (5, 102).

There has always been a considerable interest in the morphological substrates of memory; and in the course of systematic studies it was revealed that anticholinergic drugs which produce consciousness disturbance (delirium), such as atropine, hyoscine, and Ditran®, impair acquisition and retention in animals, while cholinergic substances, such as diisopropylfluorophosphate and physostigmine, exert an opposite effect. In subsequent human pharmacological studies it was revealed that physostigmine reversed the scopolamine or Ditran® induced memory disturbance. The findings that physostigmine, a cholinergic agent, reversed the impairment of memory storage and retrieval indicates that the memory dysfunction induced by scopolamine and Ditran® may be related to the cholinergic blockade produced by these drugs. In favor of the hypothesis that cholinergic agonists may have a favorable effect on memory are the findings that intravenous administration of physostigmine, in the dosage of 1 mg, significantly enhanced the storage of information in normal subjects, while intravenous administration of physiological saline did not; that parenteral administration of arecoline, a cholinergic agonist, in the dosage of 4 mg, and choline, a precursor of acetylcholine, significantly enhanced serial learning in normal subjects; that the scopolamine (0.5 mg) induced impairment of learning was reversed by the subsequent injection of arecoline; and that small 0.8 mg doses of physostigmine, given subcutaneously, produced favorable changes in memory and cognitive functions in 13 aged individuals (27, 29, 34, 35, 119).

Independent from this line of research, in a series of systematic studies in which animals were either rotated on a turntable, trained to balance on a steel wire, or trained to transfer handedness, it has been revealed that sensory stimulation gives rise to increased synthesis of RNA in the involved nerve cells without a change in the proportion of adenine (A) and uracil (U). On the other hand, establishment of new behavior was found to be associated with an increase in the A/U ratio. Furthermore, the synthesis of two acidic protein fractions—with a molecular weight of 30,000—increased by 100 percent in the hippocampal nerve cells during a learning experiment carried out in rats. The newly synthesized exclusive brain proteins are characterized by a high percentage of glutamic acid and aspartic acid content and by the virtual lack of tryptophan. On the basis of his findings, Hyden (67) put forward the notion that learning involves an increase in the synthesis of messenger RNA (mRNA), with a highly specific base composition, and the synthesis of certain specific acidic protein fractions, the biochemical substrates of long-term memory.

Independent of its scientific merit, Hyden's (67) speculation prompted Cameron and Solyom (19) to administer yeast RNA to geriatric patients with memory disturbance. As a result, in uncontrolled and placebo-controlled studies they found the investigational substance to be therapeutically effective in the treatment of senile and arteriosclerotic dementia. But subsequent studies with labeled RNA, carried out by the same group of investigators revealed that the RNA molecules did not enter into the cerebral neurons. They could only be found in the cells of the ependyma of the the plexus choroideus. In view of this, it was suggested that the therapeutic effects that had been observed with RNA were due to one of the breakdown products of RNA, which was thought to have increased the endogenous RNA content of cerebral neurons. Similar speculations led to the development of substances with a facilitating effect on RNA synthesis. Among these substances magnesium pemoline received the most publicity. Nevertheless, the initial favorable results with magnesium pemoline could not be confirmed in subsequent clinical investigations. More recently, Droller, Bevans, and Jayaram (36), in an eight week, double-blind, cross-over clinical trial, with a group of 22 elderly women, found that pemoline had no therapeutic advantage over an inactive placebo. Besides magnesium pemoline, there is only one other RNA stimulating substance, tricyanoaminopropene, which has been explored clinically. While tricyanoaminopropene may facilitate RNA synthesis and improves learning as well as short term memory in animals it has no therapeutic effect in man (3, 20, 72, 78, 79, 106, 125).

While Hyden (67) has considered that certain specific acidic proteins are the biochemical substrates of long-term memory, other investigators put forward the notion that the biochemical basis of memory lies in protein synthesis. No corresponding investigations in humans, however, have been carried out in this particular area of research (3, 9, 23, 43, 44, 71).

Simultaneously with the steadily accumulating information on the role of protein synthesis and breakdown, some evidence has been given that neuropeptides may also have an influence on memory functions. Accordingly, in a series of systematic studies it was possible to show that administration of the pituitary hormone β-lipotropin (β-LPH), the adrenocorticotropin hormone peptide, ACTH 4-10 (a peptide whose amino acid sequence is identical to β-LPH 47-53), the neurohypophyseal hormone vasopressin, and two naturally occurring penta-peptides, leucine-enkephalin and (especially) methionine-enkephalin (β-LPH 61-65), have attenuated experimentally induced amnesia in rats. Furthermore, while

82

the peptide hormone ACTH 4-10 restored the impairment of acquisition, and the unusually rapid extinction of the conditional avoidance reflex in hypophysectomized rats, implantation of glucocorticoid hormones, such as corticosterone or dexamethasone into various regions in the ascending reticular system, or the limbic forebrain, exerted an action opposite to that induced by ACTH 4-10. From a clinical point of view, however, most important are the findings that in preliminary studies at least two of these neuropeptides, ACTH 4-10 and vasopressin, were found to improve learning and memory functions. If these findings could be substantiated by further clinical experiments, memory research in the aged would enter into a new phase (4, 30, 31, 46, 71, 111).

B. Dementia

Research efforts to identify the morphological substrates of dementia yielded limited success. Since the weight of the human brain gradually decreases after middle age, a weight differential of 9 to 11 percent in brain volume (relative to skull capacity) is considered to be within normal range, and only changes above 12 percent indicate atrophy. The decrease of brain volume is due, only in part, to cerebral infarctions, present in approximately 50 percent of normal subjects above 65 years of age. Considerably more important is that during the normal life span, there is a loss of approximately 20 percent of cerebral neurons. The decrease of neurons is preceded by the destruction of cellular components (lysosomes by free radicals), deterioration of enzymatic activity, and deposition of metals or pigment bodies (lipofuscin), and is associated with a decrease of synaptic contacts. Nevertheless, whether the loss of neurons is responsible for the mild to moderate mental dysfunction seen in more than 10 percent of those 65 years or older has remained undecided to date (16, 17, 33, 54, 73, 77, 128, 133).

New structural elements, such as senile plaques and neurofibrillary tangles (also granulo-vacuolar degeneration and Hirano bodies) appear in the human brain with aging. While senile plaques are microscopic lesions with a central amyloid core surrounded by a less densely staining fibrillary or granular zone, neurofibrillary tangles consist of intraneural fibrils that have become thickened, twisted, and distorted within the neuronal perikaryon. Both senile plaques and neurofibrillary tangles start to appear in middle age and gradually increase with age.. Although they are present in approximately 70 percent of all people over 65, a positive relationship between the number of senile plaques and/or neurofibrillary tangles and the severity of dementia has been revealed. In fact, the density of senile plaques in normal (aged) brains rarely exceeds 14 per low-power microscopic field (1.3 mm in diameter) and only in the brains of patients with dementia do they invade all cortical layers (13, 40, 54, 133).

It has been noted that glucose utilization, total lipid concentration, the incorporation of amino acids into protein, and total protein levels are decreased in the aged human brain. Nevertheless, no relationship between these changes and the severity of dementia could be revealed (33).

In spite of the insufficient evidence of a relationship between decreased glucose utilization and dementia, Funfgeld (47) has decided to treat patients suffering from chronic diffuse cerebrovascular and metabolic processes with actihaemyl, a protein-free extract obtained from the blood of young calves, which assumedly increases glucose utilization in the brain. As a result, 57 percent of his patients improved within two to four weeks. He was similarly successful with pyritinol, also referred to as pyrithioxine, a substance which has been shown to increase glucose utilization and decrease adrenaline-induced lipolysis in aged psychiatric patients. Furthermore, in a psychometric study, pyritinol improved performance in a short-term attention task. Most important, however, are the findings of a recent clinical study in moderate to severe organic brain syndrome patients in which pyritinol in the dosage of 600 mg per day produced significantly greater improvement than an inactive placebo in activity, alertness, mental power, and interest, after six to nine weeks of treatment (10, 47, 62, 115).

A functionally, but not structurally related substance to pyritinol is naftidrofuryl, which has been shown to improve cerebral glucose utilization, intellectual performance, and short-term memory. If these findings could be borne out by further clinical evidence, pyritinol and naftidrofuryl would become important pharmacological agents in the treatment of dementia (14, 15, 94).

V. DIAGNOSTIC TECHNIQUES

Since the same etiology may result in a variety of psychopathological symptoms and similar psychopathological symptoms may result from a variety of etiologies, a careful psychiatric history and psychopathological assessment has to be supplemented with ancillary diagnostic techniques for diagnostic accuracy. The basic routine diagnostic battery for patients with possible organic brain disease according to Wells (133) should include urinalysis, chest X-ray, blood studies (complete blood count, serological test for syphilis, standard metabolic screening battery, serum thyroxine by column, vitamin B_{12} and folate levels), and computerized tomography.

A. Computerized Tomography

While laboratory tests may be instrumental in the diagnosis of extracerebral etiologies, neuroradiological techniques play an important role in the identification of the site and size of brain lesions in geropsychiatric patients. Nevertheless, because of the limited information it provides, plain skull X-ray should be supplemented by brain scanning (isotope encephalography) and RISA (radioactive iodinated human serum albumin tagged with ^{131}I) encephalography. Somewhat different information is provided by carotid or vertebral angiography, and lumbar, cysternal, or ventricular pneumography. Since enlargement of the cerebral ventricles and of the subarachnoid space occurs in ordinary senescence in a rather high percentage of patients without dementia, pneumoencephalography plays a more important role in the investigation of presenile, than senile dementia. There are indications that pneumography is being increasingly replaced by tomography and positive contrast ventriculography which provides for a better visualization of the ventricular system.

Computerized tomography (CT) is a new method of visualizing cerebral structures including the ventricular system and cortical sulci. It consists of the acquisition of information from different views within a single cross-sectional plane, and the computation of these data to present a recognizable image. The brightness of each portion of a cross-section of the brain in the final image is proportional to the degree to which it absorbs X-rays. By employing CT it was revealed that geropsychiatric patients with moderate or severe cerebral atrophy had a poorer short-term prognosis than geropsychiatric patients with mild atrophy. Furthermore, in a recently conducted study CT proved to be a simple and practical screening procedure for patients with senile dementia (1, 45).

Since the introduction of a new class of nootropic drugs, early recognition of cerebral atrophy or other changes which may lead to personality deterioration has become especially important. Piracetam, a 2-oxo-1-pyrrolidineacetamide, a cyclic GABA derivative, is the first member of this new class of psychotropic drugs, which

Psychotropic Drug Research

according to Giurgea (48) act selectively on telencephalic integrative mechanisms. In animal experiments it was revealed that the new drug promotes interhemispheric transfer, protects against experimental amnesic agents, and facilitates electroencephalographic recovery after severe hypoxia with virtually no effects on autonomic functions, arousal level, limbic lobe activity, and psychomotor behavior. Corresponding with the animal pharmacological data are the results of human pharmacological studies in which piracetam in the dosage of 4800 mg per day was shown to produce significant improvement in mental performance, and direct and delayed recall of verbal learning. Furthermore, experimental results in human subjects with artificial pacemakers indicate that piracetam counteracts the cognitive impairment due to hypoxia, induced by the slowing of the pacemaker rate. Most important, however, are the results of a controlled, double-blind clinical study in which piracetem produced significantly greater improvement in the general mental condition and behavior of organic brain syndrome patients than an inactive placebo. In another controlled clinical study in a group of elderly persons complaining of failing memory, Mindus et al (96) found that piracetam produced significant beneficial effects on mental tasks demanding vigilance, while placebo did not. In none of these studies were side effects observed. Could these findings be further substantiated by clinical evidence, piracetam would become an important drug in the prevention and treatment of dysmnesia and dementia in the aged. While the action mechanism of piracetam is unknown, Nicholson, and Wolthuis (100, 101) suggested that it selectively activates brain adenylate kinase, an enzyme facilitating ATP formation under anaerobic conditions, and inhibits cortical release of proline, a putative inhibitory neurotransmitter. Confirmation of these findings would provide a starting point for the understanding of the mechanism of action of nootropic drugs (32, 49, 82, 86, 113, 122, 132).

B. Regional Cerebral Blood Flow

Among the various new diagnostic methods one of the most important is the measuring of regional cerebral blood flow (rCBF) by employing an isotope clearance technique. The rCBF technique is based on the recognition that above a critical perfusion pressure of about 60 mm Hg the blood flow of the brain is ultimately regulated by the metabolism of the nervous tissue. While the classical nitrous oxide technique provided evidence of a positive correlation between

86

the global functional state of the brain, its blood flow and oxidative metabolism, the rCBF technique has brought to attention that regional alterations of cerebral circulation are caused by local metabolic events related to the neuronal activity of mentation (69).

Systematic studies revealed a relationship between cerebral blood flow and dementia. While normal aging appears to produce little or no change in cerebral blood flow or oxygen uptake, in cerebral arteriosclerosis both cerebral blood flow and oxygen uptake are reduced. The reduction was found to be more marked in patients with dementia. Furthermore, it has also been revealed that the functional level of the dominant hemisphere, measured by (mean hemisphere) rCBF correlates with the cognitive ability of patients with presenile dementia. Loss of neurons and degenerative changes were found in patients showing defects of symbol processing on a general level, and the defect was more pronounced when the flow reduction was severe. In addition, certain rCBF abnormalities correlate with specific cognitive functions. Accordingly, patients with memory disturbance only, demonstrated a focal flow reduction in the temporal region, while more severely affected patients, with reduction of verbal abilities and agnosia, showed very low flows also in the occipito-temporo-parietal areas. From a psychopathologic point of view, however, most important are the findings that in patients with presenile dementia, the depression anxiety syndrome is associated with a lowered mean overall rCBF, hypochondriac-hysteroid traits with relatively high rCBF in the frontal lobes, paranoia with low flow in the temporo-occipital region, affective lability among the least cognitively impaired patients with high flow in the upper frontal and premotor regions, and among the most deteriorated patients with low flow in the lower frontal region, explosive-restlessness with high flow in the motor area and low flow in the frontal region, and psychomotor overactivity with low flow in the frontal region and high flow in the postcentral areas (52,53,55, 104,118).

Development of the rCBF technique revived interest in cerebral vasodilators in geropsychiatric practice. These drugs are employed on the basis of the assumption that the psychopathology of cerebral arteriosclerosis is the result of neuronal damage produced by reduced cerebral blood flow. Nevertheless, the fact remains that cerebral blood flow is significantly reduced in geropsychiatric patients with cerebral arteriosclerosis, regardless of the presence of psychopathology. It seems that it is the decrease in cerebral oxygen consumption which indicates organic brain syndrome (121).

Psychotropic Drug Research

Whether or not cerebral vasodilators can overcome the chronic state of hypoxia produced by the reduced cerebral blood flow in cerebral arteriosclerosis has remained an open question. Sathananthan and Gershon (114) argue that factors that cause vasodilation, such as autoregulation, lactosis, and decrease in pH, in and around the ischemic areas, have already exerted their maximal vasodilating effect by the time of cerebral vasodilator administration. It has also been considered that the healthy parts of the brain receive extra blood by the dilation of the healthy vessels ("intracerebral steal syndrome"), and because of the differences in perfusion pressure shunt blood away from the ischemic areas under the influence of vasodilator drugs. But even if the ischemic areas would obtain increased blood flow, the increase in the blood supply might be in excess ("luxury perfusion syndrome") of the metabolic demands.

Irrespective of these considerations, there have been several cerebral vasodilators tested clinically during the past decade in the treatment of geropsychiatric patients, with demonstrable therapeutic effects. Carbon dioxide is one of the most potent cerebral vasodilators. Nevertheless, there is no evidence that inhalation of carbon dioxide (CO_2) has any therapeutic effect in cerebral arteriosclerosis. On the other hand, there are indications that the immediate response to the administration of 5 percent CO_2 and 95 percent oxygen may serve as a predictor of therapeutic responsiveness to specific drugs in geropsychiatric patients. Accordingly, Lehmann and Ban (88) reported that a favorable therapeutic response to nicotinic acid was associated with an overall increase in psychometric test performance following a pharmacological load of CO_2 and impaired test performance following a pharmacological load of methamphetamine. These observations, however, must be confirmed. Since prolonged treatment with CO_2 inhalation is impractical, the possibility was raised that the administration of acetazolamide (1000 to 2000 mg per day), a carbonic anhydrase inhibitor which produces cerebral vasodilation by increasing CO_2 concentration, may be a suitable alternative. Nevertheless, while the increase in cerebral blood flow, after intravenous acetazolamide administration, has been substantitated in both animal and man, acetazolamide has not become an effective therapeutic agent in the treatment of cerebral arteriosclerosis because habituation develops to its vasodilating effects within a few days (8,84, 110,114).

Sustained release papaverine is one of the most widely prescribed cerebral vasodilators. Nevertheless, the possibility that the therapeutic action of papaverine (600 mg per day) is due to phosphodiesterase inhibition, or dopamine receptor blockade, rather than to cerebral vasodilation should not be ignored. Cyclandelate shows structural similarities to papaverine. It resembles papaverine also in its action mechanism and side effects. Nevertheless, since in some of the clinical studies the statistically significant improvement in mental functions with cyclandelate (1200 to 1600 mg per day) was found to be independent from cerebral blood flow changes, Taylor (126) put forward the notion that the primary action of cyclandelate might be on cerebral metabolism and not on cerebrovascular tone. Or, in other words, the demonstrated increase in cerebral blood flow might be the result, rather than the cause of improvement in metabolism and cerebral function under the influence of the drug (103, 116).

In contrast to papaverine and cyclandelate, which have an effect on both normal and arteriosclerotic brains, there are indications that the nicotinic acid-induced increase in blood flow is restricted to patients with cerebral arteriosclerosis. Among the other vitamins, tocopherol, or vitamin E, has been implicated in having vasodilating properties. There is no conclusive evidence, however, that tocopherol improves cerebral blood flow and/or arteriosclerotic dementia to date (38, 50, 88, 114).

Among the various other mechanisms that may result an increase in cerebral blood flow is a β-receptor stimulation; and there are at least two structurally related drugs, isoxsuprine and nylidrin, that produce cerebral vasodilation via this action. There is sufficient evidence to believe that isoxsuprine increases cerebral blood flow and fulfills the criteria of a cerebral vasodilator. The effects of nylidrine are less consistent than that of isoxsuprine. The same applies to the clinical findings in senility and cerebral arteriosclerosis which are consistently favorable only with isoxsuprine (8).

Among the various other substances with cerebral vasodilating effects are the antiserotonin substance, methysergide, lipotropic enzymes, plasma kinins (kallidin decapeptides and bradykinin-nonapeptides), and PGE_2, one of the prostaglandins. Finally there are several reports in the literature in which dicumarol, an anticoagulant, has been successfully employed in the treatment of presenile and senile dementia. However, the danger of internal bleeding with this therapy is great (8, 114, 131).

VI. CLINICAL PSYCHOPATHOLOGY

A. Arteriosclerotic Dementia

Although there are many conditions in old age in which dementia may occur, e.g., intracranial tumor, general paresis of the insane, chronic post-traumatic encephalopathy, epilepsy, chronic alcoholism, normal pressure hydrocephalus, by far the most common are three degenerative processes, referred to as arteriosclerotic dementia, Alzheimer's disease, and senile dementia. While in arteriosclerotic dementia, the degenerative changes in the blood vessels may lead to focal destruction of the brain tissue, in Alzheimer's disease and senile dementia the degenerative changes in the grey matter may lead to diffuse destruction of the cerebrum (24).

There is sufficient evidence to believe that in most cases of arteriosclerotic dementia both the large and small cerebral vessels are affected, and there are indications that the dementia becomes manifest and progresses through the occurrence of multiple small or large cerebral infarcts. At necropsy the heart is found to be usually enlarged, and death is attributable to ischemic heart disease in about 50 percent of patients (24, 54).

In a study of 50 randomly selected demented patients, Tomlinson, Blessed, and Roth (127) found that cerebral infarctions accounted for the dementia in 12 percent of their elderly subjects and contributed significantly to the clinical manifestations in another 25 percent. Arteriosclerotic dementia is more common in men than women with an average age at onset in the late sixties, although the variation from patient to patient is considerable. By the time the dementia becomes apparent there is usually a history of strokes and a legacy of them in the form of hemianopia, dysphasia, and/or hemiplegia. The course of the illness is punctuated by episodes of clouding of consciousness, associated with a variety of neurological syndromes, presumably due to fresh infarcts which are usually followed by an increase in the severity of dementia. Accordingly, there is a tendency for the dementia to fluctuate in severity, and since the destruction of the cerebral cortex is not confluent, the deterioration of personality is not very profound. This is best exemplified by the observation that the essence of the personality is often surprisingly preserved and "some insight may linger" until the terminal stage. Taking all these into consideration, prerequisites for the diagnosis of arteriosclerotic dementia are the presence of one or more of the following features: abrupt onset, stepwise deterioration, fluctuating course, history of strokes and sustained hypertension, presence of significant hypertension and focal neurologic signs (112, 127, 133, 134).

One of the most systematically studied and frequently employed drugs in the treatment of arteriosclerotic dementia is Hydergine®, a dihydrogenated ergot alkaloid, containing dihydroergocornine, dihydroergocristine, and dihydroergocryptine in equal proportions. It is an α-adrenergic receptor blocking agent, which was found to be superior to an inactive placebo in 11 and to papaverine in 5 double-blind clinical studies and its effectiveness is not restricted to one specific diagnostic group. While for some time it was thought that the therapeutic action of Hydergine® is due to the decrease in vasomotor tone and cerebrovascular resistance with a consequent improvement of cerebral blood flow and transit time, more recently it has been revealed that the drug has a considerably more complicated action mechanism. Apparently Hydergine® inhibits the breakdown of adenosine triphosphate and thereby improves the energy balance in the neuron; increases the pyruvate-lactate ratio in hypothermic and ischemic brain disease and consequently restores normal neuronal oxidation that leads to the normalization of depressed EEG energies; inhibits the enzyme phosphodiesterase, i.e., interferes with the breakdown of cyclic AMP and increases the incorporation of 3H-leucine into rat brain. All these findings suggest that Hydergine® may have direct metabolic, rather than purely vascular actions and that the opening of the cerebral vessels under the influence of the drug is a consequence and not the cause of increased brain metabolism. This complex action may also explain the effectiveness of Hydergine® in conditions other than arteriosclerotic dementia (7, 8, 39, 64, 116).

Besides Hydergine®, many other drugs have been tried in the treatment of arteriosclerotic dementia. Hall and Harcup (56) observed some improvement in subjective complaints of depression and lack of energy with lipotropic enzymes, a mixture of citrogenase, amino acid oxidase and tyrosinase. Other attempts to treat the disorder included the administration of β-glucuronidase, cytochrome C, and catalase. Young, Hall, and Blakemore (136) in a long-term (12 month), controlled cross-over clinical trial found the vasodilator substance, cyclandelate (in the daily dosage of 1600 mg) significantly superior to an inactive placebo in arresting the decline of patients. Overall performance, comprehension, and vocabulary were significantly better while on active treatment. Whether other cerebral vasodilators, or drugs, such as pyrithioxine and naftidrofuryl, which produce an increase in glucose utilization, will have favorable therapeutic effects, remains to be seen (2, 8, 66, 74, 85).

B. Senile Dementia

The most striking, but inconsistent biological feature of senile dementia is the senile plaque which consists of an argyrophilic core surrounded by a clear halo with an outer peripheral ring of granular or filamentous argyrophilic material. Another and probably more consistent change is the neurofibrillary degeneration of nerve cells, that consists of bundles of microtubules, constricting and twisting, which produce in the cytoplasma a tangled mass, the neurofibrillary tangle. In senile dementia, the patient virtually vanishes away, and at necropsy, not only the brain, but also the rest of the body and the viscera are small and atrophied (24, 60).

In contrast to cerebral arteriosclerosis, senile dementia is more common in women than in men, with an average age at onset in the early seventies. By the time the dementia becomes apparent there is usually a history of episodes in which the patient is inattentive, fuddled, and frightened. Not infrequently, the patient misperceives surroundings, expresses ill-formed and poorly sustained delusions of persecution, and wanders away from home. In a controlled study Waldton (130) found a significantly greater and faster decrease in olfactory functions in patients with senile dementia than in aged-matched normal subjects. Regression of the gustatory function was slower than of the olfactory function in patients, while it was absent entirely in the controls. The same applied to auditory impairment. Although the onset of the illness may be gradual, once it is established, it advances rapidly, bringing about a profound deterioration of memory, intellect, and personality, with total dissolution of personality. About 58 percent of all patients with a diagnosis of senile dementia are dead within six months of admission, as compared to only 33 percent of all patients with a diagnosis of arteriosclerotic dementia. Since there are indications that this extremely serious and deadly disease follows a dominant or multifactorial mode of transmission with a four times greater risk for the relatives than the risk in the general population, it is expected that there will be a considerable increase in the number of patients with senile dementia because of the rapid increase in average life expectancy at birth (11, 83, 107, 112).

There is no accepted treatment of senile dementia to date. Most recently, however, deanol (2-dimethylaminoethanol), a substance which is assumed to increase brain acetylcholine (in the daily dose of 1800 mg), was found to produce overall improvement in 10 of 14 patients with senile dementia over a four-week period. However, neither the clinical ratings nor an extensive pre- versus post-treatment series of cognitive tests revealed changes in memory or other cognitive functions. The favorable action was due to improvement of depression, anxiety, irritability, motivation, and initiative. Since a similar study with a different compound produced no behavioral changes in a similar population, Ferris et al (42) assert that "it is unlikely that the improvement with deanol was due entirely to placebo effects." Other substances which produced favorable changes in senile dementia include the nootropic drug, piracetam, and ACTH 4-10, the hepta-peptide fragment of the adrenocortico-tropic hormone. Whether any one of these therapeutic approaches will succeed remains to be seen (5, 6, 31, 49).

C. Alzheimer's Disease

Since neuropathological and clinical changes in Alzheimer's disease are virtually indistinguishable from those seen in senile dementia, it has been suggested that onset before 65 signifies Alzheimer's disease and onset after 65, senile dementia. Nevertheless, Heston (60) revealed that only the relatives of patients with Alzheimer's disease have excessive incidences of trisomy 21, myeloprol-iferative disorders, and hematologic malignancies. On the basis of these findings he raised the possibility of a genetic diathesis in Alzheimer's disease which is distinctly different from that of senile dementia. This of course, corresponds with Larsson's (83) findings that the morbidity risk for senile dementia but not for Alzheimer's disease, is 4.3 times greater in the siblings than in the general population (61, 75, 76).

Biochemical investigations revealed that homovanillic acid (HVA) values in the lumbar spinal fluid are significantly lower in patients with Alzheimer's disease, than in age matched controls, and after probenecid loads increased significantly less than in patients with cerebral arteriosclerosis. On the other hand, lactate-pyruvate ratios were found to be significantly higher among Alzheimer patients than in controls. Systematic neurochemical studies brought to attention the decrease in total protein and increase in total lipid, resulting in a decreased protein-lipid ratio in the grey matter of deceased Alzheimer patients. Furthermore a novel protein band (enriched fraction band) with an estimated high molecular weight was found in a subfraction of isolated neurons of the hippocampal cortex (51, 68, 93, 124).

Independent of genetic considerations there are three main hypotheses concerning the underlying disease process in Alzheimer's disease: neurotoxic effect of a common environmental agent aluminum, an incomplete or unconventional viral infection, and a disorder of the immune system. Insofar as the "aluminum hypothesis" is concerned several observations have suggested that this trace metal may be toxic to the neurons and induces the formation of neurofibrillary tangles similar but not identical to those found in Alzheimer disease. Most important, however, is that the brains of patients with Alzheimer's disease contain higher concentrations of aluminum than of other geropsychiatric patients (25, 26, 76).

The possibility that slow-acting viruses may be involved in the genesis of Alzheimer's disease is based on the findings that the Alzheimer type of neurofibrillary degeneration in the cerebral cortex has been reported in two types of slow viral infections, i.e., progressive multifocal leukoencephalopathy (where alteration in the immune system of the host permits the proliferation of an otherwise benign virus), and subacute sclerosing panencephalitis (where the incomplete suppression of a measles-like paramyxovirus permits slow replication of the agent and destruction of oligodendlia resulting in progressive demyelination). Other findings in favor of the slow virus hypothesis are the identification of senile plaques in the brains of patients who died of subacute spongioform virus encephalopathies, such as kuru and Creutzfeldt-Jakob disease. The fact that amyloid, the primary constituent of senile plaques contains immunoglobulin, and may even be derived from immunoglobulins, suggests the presence of an abnormal antigen in the brains of patients with Alzheimer's disease (25, 70, 76, 90).

In spite of the steadily accumulating information on the neurochemical changes in patients with Alzheimer's disease and hypotheses about its etiology, no meaningful advances have been made in the treatment of this condition during the past years. However, on the basis of the assumption that Alzheimer's disease belongs to the group of collagen diseases with autoimmune factors playing a role in its etiology, Chynoweth and Foley (21) employed steroid hormones in the treatment of three Alzheimer patients. As a result,they found that after intramuscular hydrocortisone administration all three patients improved. So far their results have not been confirmed (86).

VII. CONCLUSIONS

1. The rapid increase in individuals over 65 years in the general population has directed attention to gerontology.
2. The high incidence of psychiatric morbidity in old people created the need for geropsychiatry.

Psychopharmacology in Geropsychiatry

3. The approximately fourfold increase in average life expectancy during recorded history has been exclusively due to disease control.
4. None of the present theories of aging have been sufficiently substantiated.
5. Average life span has been extended into a period of the life cycle where physical and psychological changes take place, which may seriously interfere with everyday functioning.
6. In spite of the considerable progress made in the pharmacological manipulation of nighttime behavior, daytime activities, and sexual functioning, the fact remains that even securing restful sleep still remains a problem in the aged.
7. Certain psychopathological symptoms and syndromes, such as dysmnesia and dementia are more common in patients above 65 years of age.
8. No psychotropic drug with proven therapeutic efficacy in dysmnesia and dementia is clinically available to date.
9. Improvement of memory with substances which assumedly increase RNA synthesis could not be replicated.
10. The favorable effects of cholinergic substances and neuropeptides on memory functions in humans need to be further substantiated in appropriately designed clinical experiments.
11. It remains to be seen whether substances which improve glucose utilization in the brain will interfere with the progress of dementia and/or improve the behavior of demented patients.
12. New diagnostic techniques, such as computerized tomography and rCBF have provided means for the identification of homogenous geropsychiatric patient populations.
13. Whether nootropic drugs, which assumedly improve telencephalic integrative mechanisms and/or cerebral vasodilators will interfere with the progress of cerebral pathology if detected at an early stage remains an open question.
14. There is a need for systematic research to develop new drugs with a differential pharmacological profile from present psychotropic substances which will have greater specificity in the treatment of arteriosclerotic dementia, Alzheimer's disease, and senile dementia.
15. There is a need for appropriate clinical research facilities in geropsychiatry where new pharmacological agents can be tested in appropriately selected homogenous patient populations by employing advanced contemporary research methods.

Psychotropic Drug Research

REFERENCES

1. Abrams, H.L. and McNeil, B.J.: Medical implications of computerized tomography. (First of two parts). *N. Eng. J. Med.*, 298:255-261, 1978.
2. Altschul, R.: Einfluss von cyctochrom C und hämatoporphyrin auf serumcholesterin. *Z. Kreislaufforsch.* 48:844-848, 1959.
3. Appel, H.: Macromolecules and memory. In S.J. Martin and B. Kisch, (Eds.): *Enzymes in Mental Health.* Lippincott, Philadelphia, 1966.
4. Bailey, A. and Grenard, P.: Memories are made of this. *Macleans,* 91:70, 1978.
5. Ban, T.A.: Psychopathology, psychopharmacology and the organic brain syndrome. I. *Psychosomatics,* 17:77-82, 1976.
6. Ban, T.A.: Psychopathology, psychopharmacology and the organic brain syndrome. II *Psychosomatics,* 17:131-137, 1976.
7. Ban, T.A.: The treatment of depressed geriatric patients. *Am. J. Psychother.,* 32:93-104, 1978.
8. Ban, T.A.: Vasodilators, stimulants and anabolic agents in the treatment of geropsychiatric patients. In M.A. Lipton, A. DiMascio, K.F. Killam (Eds.): *Psychopharmacology - A Generation of Progress,* Raven Press, New York, 1978, pp. 1525-1534.
9. Barondes, S.H. and Cohen, H.D.,: Memory impairment after subcutaneous injection of acetoxycyloheximide, *Science,* 160:556-557, 1968.
10. Becker, K. and Hoyer, S.: Studies on cerebral metabolism during pyrithioxine treatment. *Dtsch. Z. Nervenheilkd.,* 188: 200-209, 1966.
11. Bergman, K.: The epidemiology of senile dementia. *Br. J. Psychiatry,* 125 (Special No. 9):100-109, 1975.
12. Besser, G.M. and Thorner, M.O.: Bromocriptine in the treatment of the hyperprolactinaemia - hypogonadism syndromes. *Postgrad. Med. J.,* 52 (Suppl. 1):64-70, 1976.
13. Blessed, G., Tomlinson, B.E. and Roth, M: The association between quantitative measures of dementia and of senile change in the cerebral grey matter of elderly subjects. *Br. J. Psychiatry,* 114:797-811, 1968.
14. Bouvier, J.B., Passeron, O. and Chupin, M.P.: Psychometric study of Praxilene. *J. Int. Med. Res.,* 2:59-65, 1976.
15. Branconnier, R.J. and Cole, J.O.: A memory assessment technique for use in geriatric psychopharmacology: Drug efficacy trial with naftidrofuryl. *J. Am. Geriat. Soc.,* 25:186-188, 1977.
16. Brizzee, K.R., Kaack, B., and Klara, P.: Lipofuscin: intra- and extra-neuronal accumulation and regional distribution. In J.M. Ordy, K.R. Brizzee (Eds.): *Neurobiology of Aging. Advances in Behavioral Biology,* Vol. 16, Plenum Press, New York, 1975.
17. Brody, H.: Organization of the cerebral cortex. *J. Comp. Neurol.,* 102:511-556, 1955.
18. Busse, E.W.: Aging research: A review and critique. Read at American

College of Psychiatry, February, 1978, (in press).
19. Cameron, D.E. and Solyom, L.: Effects of ribonucleic acid on memory. *Geriatrics,* 16:74-81, 1961.
20. Cameron, D.E., Sved, S., Solyom, L., Wainrib, R. and Barik, H.: Effects of ribonucleic acid on memory defects in the aged. *Am. J. Psychiatry,* 120:320-325, 1963.
21. Chynoweth, R. and Foley, J.: Pre-senile dementia responding to steroid therapy. *Br. J. Psychiatry.* 115:703-708, 1969.
22. Cohen, S., Ditman, K.S., Moore, R.A. and Thorn, R.A.: The psychopharmacology of aging. *Drug Abuse and Alcoholism Newsletter,* 4: 932-947, 1975.
23. Cooper, J.R., Bloom, F.E. and Roth, R.H.: *The Biochemical Basis of Neuropharmacology,* Oxford University Press, New York, 1974.
24. Corsellis, J.A.N.: The pathology of dementia. *Br. J. Psychiatry,* 125 (Special No. 9):110-118, 1975.
25. Crapper, D.R. and DeBoni, U.: Brain aging and Alzheimer's disease. *Can. Psychiat. Assoc. J.,* 23:229-233, 1978.
26. Crapper, D.R., Kirshnan, S.S. and Dalton, A.J.: Brain aluminum distribution in Alzheimer's disease and experimental neurofibrillary degeneration. *Science,* 180:511-513, 1973.
27. Davis, K.L., Mohs, R.C., Tinklenberg, J.R., et al: Physostigmine: Improvement of long-term memory process in normal humans. *Science,* 201:272-274, 1978.
28. Denko, C.W.: Hypnotics and the geriatric patient. *Clin. Med.,* 75:27-31, 1968.
29. Deutsch, J.A.: The cholinergic synapse and the site of memory. *Science,* 174:788-794, 1971.
30. de Wied, D.: Neurohypophyseal hormones and memory. Abstracts 2nd World Congress of Biological Psychiatry, August 31-Sept. 6, 1978, pp. 27-28.
31. de Wied, D.: Pituitary-adrenal system hormones and behavior. In F. O. Schmitt, and F.G. Worden (Eds.): *The Neurosciences Third Study Program,* MIT Press, Cambridge, 1974.
32. Dimond, S.J. and Brouwers, E.Y.M.: Increase in the power of human memory in normal man through the use of drugs. *Psychopharmacologia,* (Berl.) 49:307-309, 1976.
33. Domino, E.F., Dren, A.T. and Giardina, W.J.: Biochemical and neurotransmitter changes in the aging brain. In M. Lipton, A. DiMascio and K.F. Killam (Eds.): *Psychopharmacology - A Generation of Progress,* Raven Press, New York, 1978.
34. Drachman, D.A.: Central cholinergic system and memory. In M. A. Lipton, A. DiMascio and K.F. Killam (Eds.): *Psychopharmacology - A Generation of Progress,* Raven Press, New York, 1978.
35. Drachman, D.A. and Leavitt, J.: Human memory and the cholinergic system. *Arch. Neurol.,* 30:113-121, 1974.
36. Droller, H., Bevans, H.S. and Jayaram, V.K.: Problems of a drug trial

Psychotropic Drug Research

(pemoline) on geriatric patients. *Gerontol. Clin.*, 13:269-276, 1971.
37. Dublin, L.I., Lotka, A.J. and Spiegelman, M.: *Length of Life*, Ronald Press, New York, 1949.
38. Ehrenreich, D.L., Burns, R.A., Alman, R.W. and Fazekas, J.F.: Influence of acetazolamide on cerebral blood flow, *Arch. Neurol.*, 5:227-232, 1961.
39. Emmenegger, H. and Meirer-Ruge, W.: The action of Hydergine on the brain: a histochemical, circulatory and neurophysiological study, *Pharmacology*, 1:65-78, 1968.
40. Farmer, P.M., Peck, A. and Terry, R.D.: Correlations among numbers of neurotic plaques, neurofibrillary tangles and the severity of senile dementia, *J. Neuropathol. Exp. Neurol.*, 35:367, 1976.
41. Feinberg, I. and Carlson, V.R.: Sleep variables as a function of age in man, *Arch. of Gen. Psych.*, 18:239-245, 1968.
42. Ferris, S.H., Sathananthan, G., Gershon, S. and Clark C.: Senile dementia; treatment with deanol, *J. Am. Ger. Soc.*, 25:241-244, 1977.
43. Flexner, L.B., Flexner, J.B. and Roberts, R.B.: Memory in mice analyzed with antibiotics, *Science*, 155:1377-1383, 1967.
44. Flood, J.F. Bennett, E.L., Orme, A.E., et al: Memory: modification of anisonycin-induced amnesia by stimulants and depressants, *Science*, 199:324-326, 1978.
45. Fox, J.H., Topel, J.L. and Huckman, M.S.: Use of computerized tomography in senile dementia, *J. Neurol. Neurosurg. and Psychiat.*, 38:948-953, 1975.
46. Frederiksen, S.D.: The antidysmnesic effect of ACTH 4-10. A preliminary study. Abstracts 2nd World Congress of Biological Psychiatry, August 31-Sept. 6, 1978, p. 100.
47. Fungeld, E.W.: Ergebnisse medikamentoser therapie die alterenpatienten mit cerebral-organischen storungen, *Nervenarzt*, 41:352-354, 1970.
48. Giurgea, C.: The "nootropic" approach to the pharmacology of the integrative activity of the brain, *Cond. Reflex*, 8:108-115, 1973.
49. Giurgea, C. and Salama, M.: Nootropic drugs. *Prog. Neuro-Psychopharmac.*, 1:235-247, 1977.
50. Gotoh, F., Meyer, J.S., and Tomita, M.: Carbonic anhydrase inhibition and cerebral venous blood gases and ions in man. Demonstration of increased oxygen availability to ischemic brain. *Arch. Int. Med.*, 117:39-46, 1966.
51. Gottfries, C.G., Kjallgrist, A., Ponten, V., et al: Cerebrospinal fluid pH and monoamine and glucolytic metabolites in Alzheimer's disease. *Br. J. Psychiatry*, 124:280-287, 1974.
52. Gustafson, L. and Hagberg, B.: Dementia with onset in the pre-senile period. Part II. Emotional behavior, personality changes and cognitive reduction in pre-senile dementia: Related to regional cerebral blood flow. *Acta Psychiat. Scand.* , 257 (Suppl.):37-71, 1975.
53. Gustafson, L. and Riseberg, J.: Regional cerebral blood flow related to

psychiatric symptoms in dementia with onset in the presenile period. *Acta Psychiat. Scand.* , 50:516-538, 1974.

54. Hachinski, V.C., Lassen, N.A. and Marshall, J.: Multi-infarct dementia: a cause of mental deterioration in the elderly. *Lancet*, 1:207-209, 1974.

55. Hagberg, B. and Ingvar, D.H.: Cognitive reduction in presenile dementia related to regional abnormalities of cerebral blood flow, *Br. J. Psychiatry*, 128:290-292, 1976.

56. Hall, P. and Harcup, M.: A trial of lipotropic enzymes in atheromatous (arteriosclerotic) dementia. *Angiology*, 205:287-300, 1969.

57. Hamouz, W.: Use of pyritinol in patients with moderate to severe organic psychosyndrome. *Pharmacotherapeutica*, 1:398-404, 1977.

58. Hartman, E., Chung, R. and Chien, C.P.: L-tryptophane and sleep, *Psychopharmacologia*, 19:114-127, 1971.

59. Hayflick, L.: Human aging in 2025 AD. A prospective analysis. In *Aging in America's Future.* Symposium: Dedication of the Pharmaceutical Research Center and Medical Administration Building, Hoechst-Roussel Pharmaceuticals, Inc., Somerville, New Jersey, November 7, 1975.

60. Heston, L.L.: Alzheimer's disease, trisomy 21 and myeloproliferative disorders: Association suggesting genetic diathesis, *Science*, 196:322-323, 1977.

61. Heston, L.L. and Mastri, A.R.: The genetics of Alzheimer's disease. Associations with hematologic malignancy and Dawn's Syndrome. *Arch. Gen. Psych.*, 34:976-981, 1977.

62. Hoffman, G. and Salvendy, J.: The effect of pyrithioxine in elderly patients with cerebral changes. *Wien Z. Nervenheilkd.*, 26:279-284, 1968.

63. Hollister, L.E.: *Clinical Pharmacology of Psychotherapeutic Drugs*, Churchill Livingston, New York, 1978.

64. Hollister, L.E.: Drugs for mental disorders of old age. *J.A.M.A.*, 234:195-198, 1975.

65. Hun, N.: The importance of social care in the aged. In I. Tariska (Ed.): *Neuropsychiatric Disorders in the Aged*, Medicina, Budapest, 1967.

66. Hunter, J.D.: Nicotinic acid therapy in patients with coronary disease. *N.Z. Med. J.*, 59:280-285, 1960.

67. Hyden, H.: The question of molecular basis of memory. In D.E. Broadbent (Ed.): *Biology of Memory*, Academic Press, New York, 1970

68. Igbal, K., Visniewski, M., Shelanski, M., et al: Protein changes in senile dementia. *Brain Res.*, 77:337-340, 1974.

69. Ingvar, D.H. and Lassen, N.A.: Cerebral blood flow and cerebral metabolism. *Triangle*, 9:234-243, 1970.

70. Ischii, T. and Haga, S.: Immunoelectron microscopic location of immunoglobulins in amyloid fibrils of senile plaques. *Acta Neuropath.* (Berl.), 36:243-249, 1976.

Psychotropic Drug Research

71. Iversen, Susan, D. and Iversen, L.L.: *Behavioral Pharmacology,* Oxford University Press, Oxford, 1975.
72. Kalinowski, L.B. and Hippius, H.: *Pharmacological, Convulsive and Other Somatic Treatments in Psychiatry,* Grunne and Stratton, New York, 1971.
73. Kanowski, S.: Senescent brain: Current status and implication in neuro-psychopharmacology. *Prog. in Neuro-Psychopharmacology,* 1: 249-256, 1977.
74. Kayatan, S.: Arteriosclerosis and β-glucuronidase, *Lancet,* 2:667-668, 1960.
75. Kent, S.: Can normal aging be explained by the immunologic theory?, *Geriatrics,* 32:112-138, 1977.
76. Kent, S.: Classifying and treating organic brain syndromes, *Geriatrics,* 32:87-96, 1977.
77. Kety, S.S.: Human cerebral blood flow and oxygen consumption as related to aging, *Res. Publ. Assoc. Res. Nerv. Ment. Dis.,* 35:31-45, 1956.
78. Kral, V.A., Solyom, L. and Enesco, H.E.: Effect of short term oral RNA therapy on the serum uric acid level and memory function in senile versus senescent subjects. *J. Amer. Ger. Soc.,* 15:364-372, 1967.
79. Kral, V.A., Solyom, L., Enesco, H., and Ledwidge, B.: Relationship of vitamin B_{12} and folic acid to memory function. *Biol. Psychiatry,* 2:19-26, 1970.
80. Kramer, M., Taube, C. and Starr, S.: Pattern of use of psychiatric facilities by the aged: Current status, trends and implications. In A. Simon and L.J. Epstein (Eds.): *Aging in Modern Society Psychiatric Research Report No. 23,* American Psychiatric Association, New York, 1968.
81. Kuhlen, R.G.: Aging and life adjustment. In J.E. Birren (Ed.): *Handbook of Aging and the Individual,* University of Chicago, Chicago, 1967.
82. Lagergren, K. and Levander, S.: A double-blind study on the effects of piracetam upon perceptual and psychomotor performance at varied heart rates in patients treated with artificial pacemakers, *Psychopharmacologia* (Berl.), 39:97-104, 1974.
83. Larsson, T.: *Age with a Future,* Munksgaard, Copenhagen, 1964.
84. Lassen, N.A.: The luxury perfusion syndrome and its possible relation to acute metabolic acidosis localized within the brain, *Lancet,* 2:1113-1115, 1966.
85. Lehmann, H.E.: Pharmacotherapy in geropsychiatric disorders: New perspectives. Read at the 5th World Congress of Psychiatry, Mexico City, Mexico, November 28-Deccember 4, 1971.
86. Lehmann, H.E.: Rational pharmacotherapy in geropsychiatry. Read at the 10th International Congress of Gerontology, Jerusalem, Israel, June 22-27, 1975.
87. Lehmann, H.E. and Ban, T.A.: Central nervous system stimulants

100

and anabolic substances in geropsychiatric practice. In S. Gershon and A. Raskin (Eds.): *Aging.* Volume 2, Raven Press, New York, 1975.

88. Lehmann, H.E. and Ban, T.A.: Pharmacological load tests as predictors of pharmacotherapeutic response in geriatric patients. In J.R. Wittenborn, S.C. Goldberg and P.R.A. May (Eds.): *Psychopharmacology and the Individual Patient,* Raven Press, New York, 1970.

89. Magnus, R.V. and Cooper, A.J.: A controlled study of Reactivan in geriatrics, *Mod. Geriatrics,* 4:270-276, 1974.

90. Mandybur, T.I., Nagpaul, A.S., Papas, Z. and Niklowitz, W.J.: Alzheimer neurofibrillary changes in subacute sclerosing panencephalitis. *Ann. Neurol.,* 1:103-107, 1977.

91. Masters, W.H. and Johnson, V.E.: Sex over sixty. *Geriat. Med. World News,* 1:74-76, 1971.

92. Mayer-Gross, W., Slater, E. and Roth, M.: *Clinical Psychiatry,* Cassell and Company Ltd., London, 1960.

93. McNamara, J.O. and Appel, S.H.: Biochemical approaches to dementia. In C.E. Wells (Ed.): *Dementia,* 2nd Edition, F.A. Davis Co., Philadelphia, 1977.

94. Meynaud, A., Grand, M. and Fontaine, L.: Effects of naftridrofuryl upon energy metabolism of the brain, *Arzneim. Forsch.,* 23:1431-1436, 1973.

95. Middleton, R.S.W.: Temazepam (Euhypnos) and chlormethiazole: A comparative study in geriatric patients, *J. Int. Med. Res.,* 6:121-125, 1978.

96. Mindus, P., Cronholm, B., Levander, S.E. and Schalling, D.: Piracetam-induced improvement in mental performance. *Acta Psychiat. Scand.,* 54:150-160, 1976.

97. Morrison, B.O. and Bernheim, E.: Chloral betaine: Evaluation of its sedative-hypnotic properties in geriatric patients. *J. Am. Ger. Soc.,* 11:439-444, 1963.

98. Mugard, J.P. and Laborit, H.: Gammahydroxybutyrate. In E. Usdin and I.S. Forrest (Eds.): *Psychotherapeutic Drugs, Part II, Applications,* Marcell Dekker, New York, 1977.

99. Neugarten, B.L.: The aged in the year 2025. In *Aging in America's Future.* Symposium: Dedication of the Pharmaceutical Research Center and Medical Administration Building, Hoechst-Roussel Pharmaceuticals, Inc., Somerville, New Jersey, 1975.

100. Nicholson, V.J. and Wolthuis, O.L.: Differential effects of the acquisition enhancing drug pyrrolidone acetamide (piracetam) on the release of proline from visual and parietal cerebral cortex in vitro. *Brain Res.,* 113:616-619, 1976.

101. Nicholson, V.J. and Wolthuis, O.L.: Effect of the acquisition enhancing drug piracetam on rat cerebral energy metabolism. Comparison with naftidrofuryl and methamphetamine, *Biochem. Pharm.* 25: 2241-2244, 1976.

102. Nyiro, Gy.: *Psychiatria,* Medicina, Budapest, 1962.

Psychotropic Drug Research

103. O'Brien, M.D.: Concluding remarks. In G. Stocker, R.A. Kuhn, P.Hall, S. Becker and E. van der Veen (Eds.): *Assessment of Cerebrovascular Insufficiency,* Georg Thieme Verlag: Stuttgart, 1971, pp. 148-149.

104. Obrist, W.D., Chivian, E., Cronquist, S. and Ingvar, D.H.: Regional cerebral blood flow in senile and presenile dementia, *Neurology,* 20: 315-322, 1970.

105. Pfeiffer, E.: Geriatric sex behavior. *Med. Asp. Hum. Sex.,* 3:19-28, 1969.

106. Plotnikoff, N.: Pemoline: review of performance. *Tex. Rep. Biol. Med.* 29:467-479, 1971.

107. Pratt, R.T.C.: The genetics of neurological disorders. *Oxford Monographs on Medical Genetics,* Oxford University Press, New York, 1967.

108. Prien, R.F.: Chemotherapy in chronic organic brain syndrome - A review of the literature. *Psychopharm. Bull,* 9:5-20, 1973.

109. Ravetz, E.: Chloral betaine in the management of mentally disturbed senile patients. *Curr. Ther. Res.,* 5:75-80, 1963.

110. Regli, F., Yamaguchi, T. and Waltz, A.G.: Cerebral circulation. Effects of vasodilating drugs on blood flow and the microvasculature of ischemic and nonischemic cerebral cortex. *Arch. Neurol.,* 24:467-474, 1971.

111. Rigter, H.: Attenuation of amnesia in rats by systematically administered enkephalins. *Science,* 200:83-85, 1978.

112. Roth, M. and Myers, D.H.: The diagnosis of dementia, *Br. J. Psychiatry,* 125: (Special 9):87-99, 1975.

113. Sara, S. and Lefevre, D.: Hypoxia-induced amnesia in one-trial learning and pharmacological protection by piracetam. *Psychopharmacological* (Berl.), 25:32-40, 1972.

114. Sathananthan, G.L. and Gershon, S.: Cerebral vasodilators: A review. In S. Gershon and A. Raskin (Eds.): *Aging,* Vol. 2, Raven Press, New York, 1975, pp. 155-168.

115. Scheffler, S.: Pyritinol in mental states in geriatrics. *Gaz. Med. Fr.,* 79:1754-1756, 1972.

116. Shader, R. and Goldsmith, G.N.: Dihydrogenated ergot alkaloids and papaverine: A status report of their effects in senile mental deterioration. In D.F. Klein and Rachel Gittleman-Klein (Eds.): *Progress in Psychiatric Drug Treatment.* Vol. 2, Brunner/Mazel, New York, 1976.

117. Silverstone, T. and Turner, P.: *Drug Treatment in Psychiatry,* Routledge & Kegan Paul, London, 1974.

118. Simard, D., Olesen, J., Paulson, O.B., et al: Regional cerebral blood flow and its regulation in dementia, *Brain,* 94:273-288, 1971.

119. Sitaram, N. and Weingartner, H.: Human serial learning: Enhancement with arecholine and choline and impairment with scopolamine, *Science,* 201:274-276, 1978.

120. Slater, E. and Roth, M.: *Clinical Psychiatry,* Tyndale and Cassell,

London, 1969.

121. Sokoloff, L.: Cerebral circulation and metabolism in the aged. In. S. Gershon and A. Raskin (Eds.): *Aging,* Vol. 2, Raven Press, New York, 1975.

122. Stegink, A.J.: The clinical use of piracetam, a new nootropic drug, *Arzneim. Forsch.,* 22:957-977, 1972.

123. Stotsky, B.A., Cole, J.O. and Tang, Y.T.: Sodium butabarbital (Butisol sodium) as a hypnotic agent for aged psychiatric patients with sleep disorders. *J. Am. Ger. Soc.,* 19:860-870, 1971.

124. Suzuki, K., Katzman, R. and Korey, S.R.: Chemical studies on Alzheimer's disease. *J. Neuropath. Exp. Neurol.,* 24:211-218, 1965.

125. Talland, G.A., Mendelson, J.H., Koz, G. and Aaron, R.: Experimental studies of the effects of tricyanoaminopropene on the memory and learning capacities of geriatric patients. *J. Psychiat. Res.,* 3:171-179, 1965.

126. Taylor, A.R.: Speculation about the site of action of cyclospasmol on cerebral metabolism. In G. Stocker, R.A. Kuhn, P. Hall, G. Becker and E. van der Veen (Eds.): *Assessment in Cerebrovascular Insufficiency,* Georg Thieme Verlag, Stuttgart, 1971, pp. 141-145.

127. Tomlinson, B.E., Blessed, G. and Roth, M.: Observations on the brains of demented old people. *J. Neurol. Sci.,* 11:205-242, 1970.

128. Tomlinson, B.E., Blessed G. and Roth, M.: Observations on the brains of non-demented old people. *J. Neurol. Sci.,* 7:331-356, 1968.

129. Wade, O.L.: Age and aging. *Br. Clin. J.,* 1:65-66, 1972.

130. Waldton, S.: Clinical observations of impaired cranial nerve function in senile dementia. *Acta Psychiat. Scand.* 50:539-547, 1974.

131. Walsh, A.C. and Walsh, B.H.: Senile and presenile dementia: further observations on the benefit of a dicumarol-psychotherapy regimen. *J. Amer. Ger. Soc.,* 20:127-131, 1972.

132. Wedl, W. and Suchenwirth, R.M.A.: Eigenwirkungen des GABA-Abkömlings Piracetam in doppelten Blindversuch bei gesunden Probanden. *Nervenarzt,* 48:58-60, 1977.

133. Wells, C.E.: Chronic brain disease: An overview. *Am. J. Psych.,* 135:1-12, 1978.

134. Wells, C.E.: Geriatric organic psychoses. *Psychiat. Ann.,* 8:57-73, 1978.

135. Williams, R., Karacan, I. and Hursch, C.J.: *EEG of Human Sleep Clinical Implications,* John Wiley and Sons, New York, 1974.

136. Young, J.D., Hall, P. and Blakemore, C.B.: Treatment of the cerebral manifestations of arteriosclerosis with cyclandelate. *Br. J. Psychiatry,* 124:177-180, 1974.

5

Receptor Sensitivity Modification (RSM) Produced By Chronic Administration Of Psychotropic Agents

ARNOLD J. FRIEDHOFF, M.D.

I. INTRODUCTION

A cell membrane receptor is a site at which a specific ligand can act, the receptor-ligand interaction resulting in one or more effects on the cell surface, within the cell membrane or within the cell itself. Membrane receptors are not, however, only static transducers of specific ligand-dependent effects, but are adaptive structures responsive to various changes in the receptor environment. In their seminal studies of denervation supersensitivity, Cannon and Rosenbleuth observed adaptive changes in receptor cells resulting from the loss of neurotransmitter secondary to degeneration of axon terminals (4). Although the mechanism was not clear at the time of these studies, we now know that certain receptor cells can adjust to changes in specific ligand supply by adjustments in the sensitivity or efficiency of the transduction mechanism.

No one cell receptor system can be said to be prototypical; however, several have been well studied and can serve, to some degree, as models for other systems. One neuronal system that has been intensively investigated is the striatal dopamine system. In the corpus striatum, dopamine terminals, originating from cell bodies in the substantia nigra, terminate on cholinergic cells. The postsynaptic dopaminergic receptors are primarily inhibitory in action. Thus release of dopamine from the presynaptic terminals results in the inhibition of acetylcholine release from the axon terminal of the postsynaptic cell.

This dopaminergic receptor system has several advantages in its use as a model of receptor-ligand interaction and as a system for study of the adaptation of receptor cells. A number of agonists and

Psychotropic Drug Research

antagonists have been identified which produce measurable effects, and a specific binding assay has been developed (5) which makes possible the study of changes in receptor density or affinity. In addition, the receptor has been found to be coupled to adenylate cyclase, this enzyme being activated as a result of receptor-ligand interaction. Finally, there are specific behavioral effects associated with activation or inhibition of the striatal dopamine system. It is thus possible to study the effects of a specific receptor-ligand interaction at the molecular, the cellular, and the behavioral level, and, as will be seen later, by changing the sensitivity of the various elements through pharmacological manipulation, further insight can be gained into the relationship of the various elements of an integrated behavioral response.

II. POSSIBLE SUPERSENSITIVITY OF CENTRAL DOPAMINE RECEPTOR CELLS IN PATHOGENESIS OF SEVERAL CONDITIONS

Various agonists and antagonists of the central dopaminergic system have been developed as pharmacological agents. This has occurred because of the fact that this system appears to be involved in the production of the symptoms of several disorders. Of particular interest is the curious relationship between Parkinsonism and psychosis, involving the central dopamine system. Parkinsonism is now believed to be, at least partly, the consequence of a central hypodopaminergic state. Extrapyramidal symptoms, secondary to neuroleptic drug treatment, result from the action of these drugs in blocking dopamine receptors.

Of particular interest to the thesis of this report are two other dopamine related syndromes, tardive dyskinesia and withdrawal dyskinesia. The former occurs in some patients who have been taking neuroleptics for a long period of time, and is characterized by mouth movements, tongue fibrillation, and often tic-like movements of the extremities, which persist for long periods of time, even if the medication is discontinued. The latter, withdrawal dyskinesia, occurs in some patients after abrupt withdrawal of neuroleptics and is characterized by the same symptoms as tardive dyskinesia, but usually disappears after a few weeks. These two conditions, appearing after prolonged blockade of dopamine receptors by antipsychotic drugs, have the characteristics of an adaptive response, which we felt was reminiscent of the adaptation observed by Walter Cannon (4), which he called denervation supersensitivity. Later, evidence will be presented from animal studies, confirming the fact that dopamine receptor supersensitivity does occur as an adaptive response to chronic blockade by neuroleptics.

Tardive dyskinesia is only one possible disorder related to supersensitivity of central dopaminergic receptor cells. This motoric disturbance is presumably localized in the striatal region of the brain. Several other psychiatric syndromes also appear to involve hyperdopaminergic states, possibly resulting from supersensitivity. It has been presumed that disorders that respond to dopamine receptor blocking agents (antipsychotic drugs) which reduce dopaminergic activity, may be caused initially by excessive dopaminergic activity. Conversely it has been proposed that antipsychotic drugs act therapeutically by reducing dopaminergic activity in conditions involving hyperdopaminergia. One such condition is schizophrenia. Hyperdopaminergia in schizophrenia could occur through several mechanisms, as for instance, increased synthesis and release of dopamine, or through blocked degradation; however, evidence of these metabolic abnormalities has not been forthcoming, despite intensive investigation.

An alternative cause of hyperdopaminergia might be supersensitivity of postsynaptic dopaminergic receptor cells, presumably in areas of the brain other than the corpus striatum. Lee and Seeman (9) have reported evidence of this in postmortem brain tissue of schizophrenics, although the possibility that these findings are drug related has not been absolutely ruled out. Another condition that may involve localized supersensitivity is Gilles de la Tourette Syndrome, and this condition is treatable by the neuroleptic, haloperidol.

If tardive dyskinesia is a clinical manifestation of dopamine receptor supersensitivity, it would be of interest to consider possible clinical analogues of subsensitivity, that is, if chronic blockade results in a compensatory increase in receptor sensitivity as a means for overcoming the blockade, does chronic overstimulation result in compensatory down regulation? One situation that appears to reflect this kind of response is the resistance to treatment that sometimes develops in patients with Parkinson's Disease after chronic L-dopa treatment. If the L-dopa treatment is stopped for 4-8 weeks, the Parkinsonism again becomes responsive to L-dopa.

Thus, several human conditions appear to result from the capacity of the dopamine receptor cell to adjust to dopamine supply by the process of receptor sensitivity modification (RSM). The evidence for these conclusions from human studies, however, is circumstantial. In a series of experiments we have attempted to determine directly whether dopamine receptors in rats are capable of bi-directional changes in sensitivity through pharmacological manipulation, and whether these changes have properties that might make them useful for therapeutic purposes.

III. DIRECT EVIDENCE FOR BI-DIRECTIONAL CHANGE IN DOPAMINE RECEPTOR SENSITIVITY AS A RESULT OF AGONIST OR ANTAGONIST TREATMENT

In a series of studies that I carried out with Rosengarten and Bonnet we have shown that chronic blockade produces an increase in dopamine receptor sensitivity and that this increase could be reversed by increasing the supply of dopamine through the administration of L-dopa (6). In those studies, Wistar rats were treated with haloperidol, 2 mg/kg/day intraperitoneally (i.p.) to produce supersensitivity of striatal dopamine receptors (3, 11, 12, 14 and 15), or with physiological saline i.p. for 28 days. Ten days after the termination of treatment, both groups of rats were divided into equal subgroups. Half of the saline group continued to receive saline (Group 1) while the other half received L-dopa 200 mg/kg/day, intramuscularly (i.m.) for 10 days (Group 4). Similarly, half of the haloperidol group received saline (Group 2), while the other half received L-dopa 200 mg/kg/day, i.m. for 10 days (Group 3). At the end of the 10 day period, all treatments were stopped to permit the elimination of residual L-dopa. On the fifth day after termination of treatment, all rats were sacrificed by decapitation, and the corpus striatum was rapidly dissected from both sides of the brain of each rat.

Dopamine binding assays were carried out in triplicate by the method of Creese et al (5) except that in our assay, the P_2 fraction of the corpus striatum was used rather than the P_1, as in the original method. In this assay ^3H-dopamine ($1 \times 10^{-8}M$) is incubated with the tissue fraction for 10 minutes at $37°C$ in presence and absence of (+) butaclamol ($10^{-5}M$). The amount of ^3H-dopamine displaced by (+) butaclamol is considered to be the amount of specifically bound ^3H-dopamine.

Dopamine stimulated adenylate cyclase activity was determined in striatal slices from each rat. The striatal preparations were incubated in Krebs-Ringer buffer containing 250 mM Ro20-1724 (phosphodiesterase inhibitor) for 10 minutes in a 95% CO_2-5% O_2 atmosphere at $37°C$. The reaction was stopped by the addition of trichloracetic acid (final concentration 10%). Cyclic AMP was determined by the protein binding method of Krueger et al (8). To determine sensitivity to apomorphine, 4 groups of rats, subjected to the same treatment paradigm, were administered a single dose of apomorphine and the severity of the stereotyped behavioral response measured (14).

In order to ascertain whether any of the administered L-dopa was present at the time of assay, 4 rats not used in the rest of the study were each given 400 microcuries of generally labelled ^{3}H-L-dopa (SA 400C/mMole) i.p. After 10 days no radioactivity could be detected in the corpus striatum.

In Figure 1 it can be seen that rats treated for 4 weeks with the dopamine blocker, haloperidol, compensated for the blockade by increasing the density of striatal dopamine receptors. From Scatchard analysis it was determined that there was no change in affinity of the receptors for dopamine. The increase in the density of dopamine receptors was associated with an increase in the activity of receptor coupled dopamine sensitive adenylate cyclase, and in the stereotyped behavioral response to apomorphine. We also have shown that the compensatory changes that occurred as the result of chronic blockade could be reversed by the chronic administration of L-dopa which served to increase the supply of dopamine.

Thus, when the dopamine receptor cell is deprived of dopamine by neuroleptic blockade, it attempts to overcome the blockade by becoming more sensitive. When it is exposed to an excess supply of dopamine the receptor cell compensates by becoming less sensitive.

We have also attempted to down regulate normosensitive dopamine receptor cells by administration of L-dopa to naive rats (Figure 1). In this last case we found a decrease in apomorphine stimulated stereotype, but neither receptor number or receptor coupled adenylate cyclase was significantly affected.

On the other hand, Mishra et al (10) have shown that the administration of L-dopa for 21 days, rather than for 10 days as in our study, will produce significant decreases in dopamine binding in naive rats.

In another series of experiments the persistance of supersensitivity produced by 4 weeks of haloperidol treatment at two dose levels is shown. In Figure 2 it can be seen that there is a rather sharp decline which begins at the time of discontinuation of treatment. However, after about 18 days the supersensitivity begins to plateau at a significant level above baseline and may persist at that level for some time. Seeman's group in earlier studies (13) have

Psychotropic Drug Research

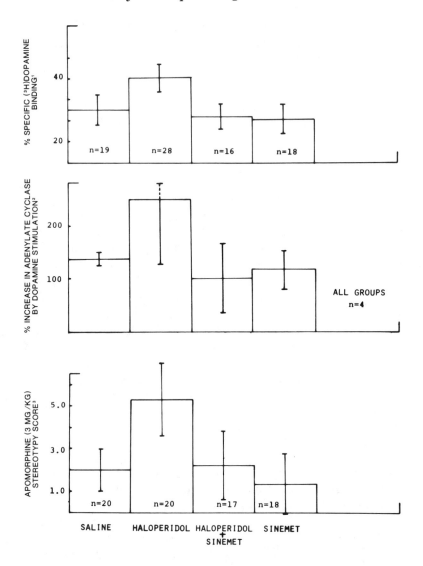

[1]Specific (³H)-dopamine binding defined as percent of total (³H) binding displaced by (+) butaclamol
[2]Adenylate cyclase activity defined as the amount of cAMP formed in 0.3mm striatal slices in the presence of Ro 20-1724
[3]Stereotypy scores were taken 30' after injection of apomorphine

FIGURE 1   Reversal of behavioral and biochemical manifestations of dopamine receptor supersensitivity by administration of sinemet (a combination of L-dopa and carbodopa).

110

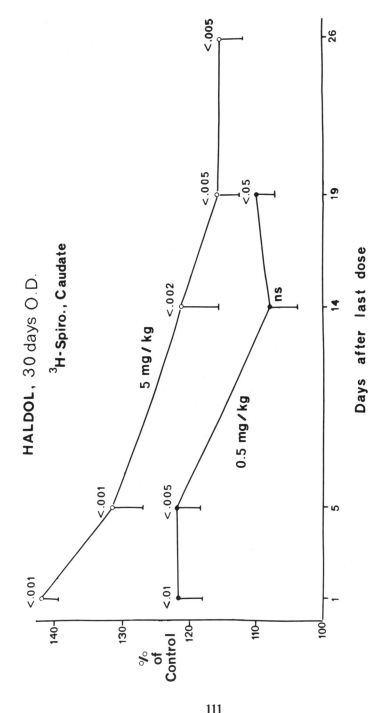

FIGURE 2

Study carried out by Jack Schweitzer, Ph.D.

reported that return to baseline after discontinuation of treatment occurs in 0.6 times the treatment period. This would coincide with the end of the period of rapid decline in our studies, but did not represent full return to baseline.

IV. RSM AS A POTENTIAL TREATMENT

As a basis for our investigation of the possibility that RSM might be useful as a treatment, we made the assumption that change in postsynaptic receptor density and/or affinity would have an effect similar to that resulting from change in agonist supply. That is:

$$\text{Response of} \atop \text{postsynaptic cell} = f \left[\begin{array}{ccc} \text{receptor} & \text{receptor} & \text{conc. of transmitter} \\ \text{density}' & \text{affinity}' & \text{at the receptor} \end{array} \right] + \begin{array}{c} \text{other} \\ \text{factors} \end{array}$$

Applying this formulation to an inhibitory striatal dopamine cell, antipsychotic drugs (dopamine receptor blockers) would acutely reduce the concentration of dopamine at the receptor by blocking its access. Thus, all other factors being equal, the inhibition of neural activity by dopamine would be decreased, and the release of acetylcholine from the axon terminal would be increased. From the data presented above, it appears that we could achieve the same result by chronic administration of L-dopa resulting in an initial increase in dopamine concentration, but an ultimate adaptive decrease in receptor density. Therefore, when L-dopa was withdrawn, there would be a decrease in the inhibitory action of dopamine and an increase in acetylcholine release. Conversely, the acute effects of dopamine agonists might be duplicated by chronic administration and then withdrawal of antipsychotic dopamine blocking drugs. Also, as is evident both from the persistence of the symptoms of tardive dyskinesia, and the data shown above in Figure 2, adaptive changes in receptors, once induced, appear to last for long periods of time after termination of drug treatment.

Thus, the basis appears to exist for utilization of the adaptive changes in the dopamine system and other similarly responding receptor systems as a novel means of pharmacological treatment, the desired therapeutic effect occurring when the treatment is stopped, and persisting for some period of time after that. In order to test the RSM approach as possible treatment, Alpert and I carried out several studies in which L-dopa (up to 6 gm/day) was administered for up to 2 months to human subjects with one of several conditions believed to involve hyperdopaminergia. In these subjects L-dopa was expected to produce an initial exacerbation of symptoms. This was, however, milder than expected. Adaptation to the L-dopa effects was observed. Some positive post-treatment effects have been noted, especially in patients with tardive dyskinesia and Gilles de la Tourette Syndrome.

V. OBSERVATIONS IN SCHIZOPHRENIA

In two studies of L-dopa in schizophrenic patients not receiving neuroleptic medication we found some initial activation followed by adaptation to the effects of the L-dopa (2, 7, 16). The activation was not in areas of primary schizophrenic signs such as thought disorder or hallucinations but, rather, in increased activity and increased expression of anger. By the end of several weeks of treatment the L-dopa treated patients were not remarkably worse than the placebo or neuroleptic treated comparison groups. Those patients who were relatively better clinically on termination of treatment with L-dopa, tended to show more activation and greater extrapyramidal involvement early in the course of treatment. Studies of the effect of L-dopa withdrawal treatment in schizophrenia are presently ongoing, and the usefulness of this treatment cannot be fully assessed at present.

VI. OBSERVATIONS IN TARDIVE DYSKINESIA

A similar dose regimen has been tried in ten patients with persisting tardive dyskinesia (1). In these studies, which are also still ongoing, we have found that most but not all patients show some increase in dyskinetic movements early in the course of treatment. Although treatment with L-dopa can exacerbate the profile of dyskinetic symptoms, it does not appear to produce a progression to new symptom involvement. About half the patients studied to date have shown a salutory response after the L-dopa treatment was terminated presumably because of a decrease in receptor number after chronic L-dopa. Their course was marked by adaption to increasingly higher doses of L-dopa and significant clinical improvement within a week or two of treatment offset.

VII. OBSERVATIONS IN GILLES DE LA TOURETTE SYNDROME

We have studied three patients with Gilles de la Tourette Syndrome who were unable to tolerate haloperidol, the present treatment of choice. With L-dopa all showed early increase in tics and vocalizations and then adaptation and improvement on treatment withdrawal. In two patients tics returned after 4-5 months and additional trials with L-dopa were attempted. In both patients, the L-dopa was much better tolerated on the second trial, while the third showed a modified course of exacerbation and adaptation with improvement after termination of treatment. One patient with a borderline adjustment showed marked delusional thinking while receiving L-dopa, and all showed evidence of transient obsessive or compulsive behaviors. These behaviors reversed when drug was withdrawn.

VIII. CONCLUSION

We have shown that modification of the sensitivity of dopamine receptor cells can be achieved by altering ligand supply. Increasing dopamine at the receptor for a prolonged period will cause a reduction in the density of receptors. Conversely, decreasing the supply of dopamine at the receptor by chronic receptor blockade will produce a compensatory increase in receptor density. These changes, once produced, persist for long periods after the termination of the treatment. These properties of the receptor system make receptor sensitivity modification (RSM) useful as a possible new approach to treatment, the therapeutic effect occurring when the pharmacological agent is discontinued. The same principle may be useful in the treatment of other neuronal or hormonal conditions that involve receptor systems subject to adaptive responses, such as insulin resistant diabetes. In these patients insulin supply is high, but the receptor nonresponsive. Administration of insulin may further down regulate the system, worsening the condition further over the long range. In contrast to this type of substitution therapy, receptor sensitivity modification uses the adaptive effect as the desired therapeutic response. The hope for the future is that these dynamic adaptive effects of the cell can be successfully manipulated so that the restitutive capacity of the organism can be maximally utilized in the treatment of disease.

References

1. Alpert, M. and Friedhoff, A.J. Clinical applications of receptor modification treatment. In R.C. Smith, W.E. Fann, J.M. Davis and E.F. Domino (Eds.), *Tardive Dyskinesia: Research and Treatment.* Spectrum Book, New York, 1978 (in press).

Receptor Sensitivity Modification

2. Alpert, M., Friedhoff, A.J., Marcos, L. and Diamond, F. Paradoxical reaction to L-dopa in schizophrenics. *Am. J. Psychiatry* 1978, (in press).
3. Burt, D.R., Creese, I., Prado, J., Croyle, J.T. and Snyder, S.H. Dopamine receptor binding: influence of age, chronic drugs and specific lesions. *Neurosci. Absts.* 2:775, 1976.
4. Cannon, W.B. and Rosenbleuth, A. *The Supersensitivity of Denervated Structures; A Law of Denervation,* MacMillan, New York, 1949.
5. Creese, I., Burt, D.R. and Snyder, S.H. Dopamine receptor binding: differentiation of agonist and antagonist states with ^{3}H-haloperidol. *Life Sci.* 17:933-1022, 1975.
6. Friedhoff, A.J., Bonnet, K.A. and Rosengarten, H. Reversal of two manifestations of dopamine receptor supersensitivity by administration of L-dopa. *Res. Comm. Chem. Path. Pharmacol.* 16:411-423, 1977.
7. Gutierrez, M., Alpert, M., Guimon, J., Friedhoff, A.J. and Veramendi, V. Investigacion farmacololgica de la funcion extrapiramidal en la esquizofrenia, *2nd World Congress of Biological Psychiatry,* Barcelona, Spain, 1978.
8. Krueger, B.K., Forn, J., Walter, J.R., Roth, R. and Greengard, P. Stimulation by dopamine of adenosine cyclic 3',5'-monophosphate formation in rat caudate nucleus. *Mol. Pharmacol.* 12:639-648, 1976.
9. Lee, T. and Seeman, P. Enhanced ^{3}H-neuroleptic binding in post-mortem schizophrenic brains. *Absts. of 8th Annual Meeting of Society for Neuroscience.* St. Louis, 1978.
10. Mishra, R.K., Wong, Y-W., Varmuza, S.L. and Tuff, L. Chemical lesion and drug induced supersensitivity of caudate dopamine receptors. *Life Sci.* 23:443-446, 1978.
11. Moore, K.E. and Thornburg, J.E. Drug-induced dopaminergic supersensitivity. *Advances in Neurology.* Vol. 9, D. Calne, T.N. Chase and A. Barbeau (Eds.), Raven Press, New York, 1975, pp. 93-104.
12. Muller, P. and Seeman, P. Increase specific neuroleptic binding after chronic haloperidol in rats. *Neurosci. Absts.* 2:874, 1976.
13. Seeman, P. Personal communication. *Psychopharmacology,* 1979, (in press).
14. Tarsey, D. and Baldessarini, R.J. Pharmacologically induced behavioral supersensitivity to apomorphine. *Nature, New Biol.* 245:262-263, 1973.
15. Tarsey, D. and Baldessarini R.J. Behavioral supersensitivity to apomorphine following chronic treatment with drugs which interfere with synaptic function of catecholamines. *Neuropharmacology* 13:927-940, 1974.
16. Veramendi, V., Alpert, M., Guimon, J., Friedhoff, A.J. and Gutierrez, M. Estudio controlado sobre la L-dopa en esquizofrenicos cronicos. *2nd World Congress of Biological Psychiatry,* Barcelona, Spain, 1978.

6

Peptides: Application to Research in Nervous and Mental Disorders

ARTHUR J. PRANGE, JR., M.D., PETER T. LOOSEN, M.D.
and CHARLES B. NEMEROFF, Ph.D.

I. INTRODUCTION

Almost ten years ago workers in the laboratories of Guillemin
(106) and Schally (246) discovered the chemical identity of thyrotropin-releasing hormone (TRH). Since then a variety of other
peptides have been identified. Some of these peptides (TRH; luteinizing hormone releasing hormone, LHRH; melanocyte stimulating hormone release inhibiting factor, MIF-I; somatotropin release inhibiting factor, SRIF, somatostatin) are hypothalamic hypo-
physiotropic hormones; they gain access to the portal venous system and influence the secretion of tropic hormones by the anterior
pituitary (106, 246). Other newly discovered peptides are widely
distributed. Some are concentrated in gut and the central nervous
system (CNS) (77, 117, 210, 263). These substances appear to have
endocrine functions in the periphery, but their CNS functions
cannot clearly be classified as hormonal unless their possible function as neurotransmitters is so considered.

The identity of certain peptides native to the anterior and posterior pituitary gland was known before the description of TRH.
The latter compounds are elaborated in brain and transported in
axons to the posterior pituitary, where they are released upon
receipt of appropriate stimuli. Recently an earlier finding has been
confirmed that an anterior pituitary hormone (adrenocorticotropic
hormone, ACTH) is localized in brain as well as in pituitary (149).
Thyroid stimulating hormone (TSH) may have a similar distribution (189).

The exploration of possible endocrine functions of newly-discov-

117

ered peptides has proceeded at a rapid rate. In parallel with this effort there has been a burgeoning interest in the behavioral effects of these substances (58, 223, 225, 227, 229). Some behavioral effects may be the indirect consequences of endocrine effects, but some appear to be direct, i.e., not endocrine-dependent. Thus, for example, LHRH facilitates sexual behavior in female rats even if they are hypophysectomized, ovariectomized, and adrenalectomized, provided appropriate hormonal replacements have been made (191, 192). The behavioral effects of peptides have been explored mainly in animals, and data pertaining to this body of work has been extensively reviewed (202, 203, 228). In the present review we shall emphasize behavioral effects and particularly the findings of human studies. It will usually be necessary, however, to summarize behavioral findings in animals to provide the background for human investigations. Our consideration of endocrine findings in man will be limited to those that pertain to administration of the peptide in question. Thus a considerable part of the neuroendocrinology literature has been omitted by design. One might, for example, be intererested in how growth hormone (GH) secretion responds to one or another challenge. Here, however, we shall limit ourselves to the effects of GH administration. In brief, we shall concern ourselves with peptides as independent variables. We shall consider only one peptide, neurotensin (NT), that has not yet been given to humans. In the section devoted to this substance we shall state the reasons for its inclusion.

II. HYPOTHALAMIC HYPOPHYSIOTROPIC HORMONES

A. Thyrotropin Releasing Hormone (TRH)

TRH (pGlu-His-Pro-NH$_2$) has been extensively tested for behavioral activity in animals. The tripeptide is active in many test systems. It appears to modify the action of several behaviorally active drugs and to exert certain independent effects, i.e., effects which do not require the presence of some other administered substance. In general, TRH tends to increase motivation and coping capacity of the organism. The tripeptide mimics many effects of amphetamine, though clear exceptions have been noted (180). Neurochemical effects are controversial, but there are data to suggest that the hormone increases both central noradrenergic and central serotonergic activity. We have reviewed these data in detail (228).

Peptides in Mental Disorders

(1) Affective Disorders

a. Behavioral Effects

In a double-blind crossover study of ten women with unipolar depression, TRH, 0.6 mg given as an i.v. bolus, produced a rapid, though brief and partial improvement. Observer and self-rating assessments showed that patients improved within a few hours and reached greatest improvement the day after treatment. Maximum improvement as measured by Hamilton's Rating Scale for Depression (112) was about 50% less than full remission. Patients tended to relapse to baseline severity within one week (220, 221).

Other investigators have addressed the problem of using TRH as an efficient remedy for depression. The results are disappointing (Tables I-IV). Generalizations about the many studies performed are difficult; size of dose, frequency and route of administration and population characteristics have varied greatly. Pecknold et al. (211), alone among all others, repeated our original experiment and obtained substantially the same results. Among the negative trials, the one performed by Kieley et al. (141) may be most instructive. They gave massive doses of the hormone to patients predicted to be poor drug responders. Although inferior to placebo, TRH was clearly active, for it produced intolerable side effects. Some patients showed evidence of hyperthyroidism. Furlong et al. (88) have suggested that differences in results might be attributed to the existence of endocrinologically distinct types of depression.

Since some treatments for depression are also useful in mania (222), it was reasonable to test TRH in the latter condition. Huey et al. (122) have reported the only trial. In a double-blind, placebo-controlled study of five euthyroid manic men they found reliable advantages for TRH (0.5 mg i.v.) as compared to saline.

b. Endocrine Effects

TRH causes the release from the anterior pituitary gland of thyroid stimulating hormone (TSH), prolactin (PRL) and, in certain conditions, growth hormone (GH) (28, 84, 176, 245). Thus the administration of the tripeptide provides the opportunity to observe not only behavioral response but endocrine responses as well. In our original report we noted that some depressed patients, all of whom were euthyroid by usual criteria, showed grossly blunted TSH responses. This finding has been confirmed by all authors who

119

TABLE I

TRH in depression: oral trials with positive results.

Authors	Dose	Patients	N	Blind	Control	Type	Results and Comments
van der Vis-Melsen and Wiener (1972)	40 mg on two occasions, then 10 mg daily	36-year-old man	1	Single	None	Impressionistic	Remarkable improvement after each dose of TRH not mimicked by placebo, TSH, or T_3
Itil et al. (1975)	100 mg daily on alternate days × 3	Various forms of depression	4	Double	Placebo capsules	Crossover	3 patients did better on TRH

TABLE II
TRH in depression: oral trials with negative results.

Authors	Dose	Patients	N	Blind	Control	Type	Results and Comments
Mountjoy et al. (1974)	40 mg daily × 7	Outpatients, mainly reactive depression; all drug failures	29	Double	Placebo capsules	Crossover	Patients showed no differential preference; kept on usual antidepressant treatment during trial
Turek and Rocha (1974)	100 mg alternate day × 3, early or late	Unipolar depression	16	Double	Placebo capsules	Crossover	Self-rating scale favored TRH, $p < 0.05$; doctors' and nurses' scales showed no differences
Huey et al. (1975)	200 mg alternate days × 3, or placebo	Male endogenous depression	5	Double	Placebo capsules	Crossover	No differential effects
Sugerman et al. (1975)	300 mg alternate days ×3 or placebo	Severe depression	16	Double	Placebo capsules	Crossover	No significant antidepressant activity

121

TABLE II (continued)

Kieley et al. (1976)	2-300 mg daily × 30	Reactive, neurotic depression	6	Double	Placebo capsules	Parallel comparison	TRH significantly inferior to placebo. Intolerable side effects. Some subjects thyrotropic
Schmidt (1977)	80 mg daily × 14	Endogenous depression	6	Double	Imipramine comparison	Parallel comparison	TRH inferior to imipramine

TABLE III
TRH in depression: intravenous trials with positive results.

Authors	Dose	Patients	N	Blind	Control	Type	Results and Comments
Prange et al. (1972)	0.6 mg bolus × 1	Unipolar depressed women	10	Double	Saline	Crossover after 7 days	Immediate partial improvement with relapse in 7 days
Kastin et al. (1972)	0.5 mg bolus daily × 3	Mixed types	5	Double	Saline	Crossover immediately upon completion of first treatment	Four patients showed marked improvement on TRH
Obiols et al. (1974)	0.6-2.8 mg daily; some patients later maintained on oral TRH 6-15 mg daily	About equal numbers of endogenous and reactive patients	156	Single	None	Impressionistic	Outcome: very good, 37; good, 39; fair, 46; null, 34; more effective in endogenous (p < 0.001)
Chazot et al. (1974)	0.4 mg slowly daily × 3	Unipolar patients	14	Single	None	Impressionistic	10 good or excellent results
	0.4 mg slowly daily × 3	Bipolar	4	Single	None	Impressionistic	2 good or excellent results

123

TABLE III (continued)

	Dose	Patients	N	Blind	Control	Design	Results
Maggini et al. (1974)	0.2 mg bolus × 1, then 0.6 mg daily × 3	Male endogenous patients	5	Single	None	Comparison with respective baseline	Statistically significant benefits of TRH limited to retardation on Hamilton scale; sleep pattern unchanged
Pecknold et al. (1976)	0.6 mg bolus × 1	Unipolar patients	6	Double	Saline	Crossover after 7 days	Results similar to Prange et al. (1972)
Lipton and Goodwin (1976)	0.6- or 1.2 mg bolus randomized with saline daily up to 14 days	Hospitalized primary depression	2	Double	Saline	Repeated crossover	Blind observer correctly detected TRH vs saline 12 of 14 times in 2 patients
Itil et al. (1975)	0.5- or 1.0 mg bolus × 1	Mixed forms of depression	9	Single	Saline	Crossover	Statistical advantage for TRH on several subscales
van den Burg et al. (1975)	0.5 mg bolus daily × 4	Endogenous depression	10	Double	Saline	Crossover	Advantage for TRH during first 2 days
van den Burg et al. (1976)	1.0 mg over 4 h × 1	Endogenous depression	10	Double	Saline	Crossover	Statistical advantage for TRH on objective rating scales

TABLE IV

TRH in depression: intravenous trials with negative results.

Authors	Dose	Patients	N	Blind	Control	Type	Results and Comments
Takahashi et al. (1973)	0.5 mg (? rate) 5-10 × during 14-21 days	Various forms of depression	14	Single	None	Impressionistic	TRH never better than imipramine in imipramine failures; imipramine usually better than TRH in patients given TRH first
	0.5 mg (? rate) × 1	Endogenous depression	10	Single	None	Impressionistic	No noticeable change in interview
Benkert et al. (1974)	0.6 mg slow × 1	Women with endogenous depression	12	Double	Saline and LHRH	Repeated crossover	No statistical difference between treatments
Chazot et al. (1974)	0.4 mg slow daily × 3	Neurotic, postpartum, and schizoid depressions	12	Single	None	Impressionistic	8 failures
Coppen et al. (1974)	0.6 mg bolus × 1	Unipolar depression	10	Double	Saline	Crossover	No statistical difference

TABLE IV (continued)

Study	Dose	Population	N	Blind	Placebo	Design	Results
Deniker et al. (1974)	1.0 mg slow; oral TRH later in some	Various forms of depression	18	Single	None	Impressionistic	Overall results negative; apparent TRH benefits in 6 of 12 bipolar patients
Dimitrikoudi et al. (1974)	0.6 mg bolus × 1 or saline	Endogenous depression	3	Single	Saline	Crossover	No reliable difference between TRH and saline
Ehrensing et al. (1974)	1.0 mg bolus daily × 3 or saline; then 1.0 mg daily × 7	Various forms of depression	8	Double then Single	Saline	Crossover	No clear differences between groups
Hollister et al. (1974)	0.6 mg bolus alternate days × 3	Various forms of depression in men	31	Double	Saline	Crossover	No reliable differences
Sorensen et al. (1974)	0.4 or 0.6 mg	Severe endogenous depression	4	Single	None	Impressionistic	TRH effect null; patients continued on standard treatment
Hall et al. (1975)	0.6 mg (? rate) daily × 4	Severe primary depression	10	Double	Saline	Parallel comparison	Differences statistically insignificant at 24 hr; thereafter all patients received ECT and/or antidepressant drugs

Evans et al. (1975)	0.6 mg (? rate) daily × 4	Mild reactive depression	20	Double	Saline	Parallel comparison	No statistical differences between treatments
Widerlov and Sjostrom (1975)	0.6 mg bolus daily × 7 or saline	Primary depression in men	10	Double	Saline	Parallel comparison	TRH advantage statistically insignificant
Lipton and Goodwin (1976)	0.6 or 1.2 mg bolus randomized with saline daily up to 14 days	Hospitalized primary depression	13	Double	Saline	Repeated crossover	Nurses unable to detect TRH efficacy on standard scales
Vogel et al. (1977)	0.6 mg (? rate) daily × 3	Women with endogenous depression	15	Double	Saline	Crossover	No statistical differences between treatments

studied more than a few patients (Table V). The one exception to this is a study by van den Burg et al. (281). Their second study contradicted their earlier one, and they pointed out that the slow infusion of TRH in their second study might have caused TSH synthesis (and subsequent release), this masking a deficient immediate release of the tropic hormone.

A substantial consensus has developed that about 25% of depressed patients show a blunted TSH response after TRH administration (see Table V). This event has not yet been convincingly linked to any demographic or subdiagnostic feature. It appears not to be the result of hyperthyroidism or even of thyroidal activation; Takahashi (267) showed that patients with *lowest* thyroid indices may show the greatest blunting. Blunting may in some patients be related to elevated cortisol; clearly elevated cortisol can dump the TSH response to TRH. Indeed, we found that TSH response was negatively related to baseline cortisol (170, 174). However, we (169), like others (47, 142, 176), have found some instances of blunting in patients in remission, when cortisol is usually normal. TSH blunting is not confined to depression; it may occur in alcoholism (171, 172). Thus two important questions emerge: can TSH blunting sometimes be a trait marker; does the phenomenon represent a biological link between some depressed and some alcoholic patients?

Possible alterations in PRL and GH response to TRH in depression are less clearly defined than the TSH response. We have reviewed these matters in detail (165, 224). In considering vagaries of TSH response to TRH in mental patients it is important to realize that it can be influenced by a variety of psychoactive drugs (154). This fact underscores the need for adequate drug washout before TRH testing; it also holds promise for clarifying central regulation of TSH response.

(2) Alcohol Withdrawal Syndrome

a. Behavioral Effects

We have employed TRH as an investigational tool in men in alcohol withdrawal syndrome (AWS) who showed secondary depression. In a double-blind study of 33 patients we compared the effects of TRH, 0.5 mg i.v., to the effects of nicotinic acid and of saline, both used as placebos (166, 168, 172). While all trends favored TRH, significant benefits from the hormone were found

TABLE V
TSH response to intravenous TRH challenge in affective disorders.

Year	Authors	N	Findings
		Depression - Positive Findings	
1972	Prange et al.	10	All responses borderline low or absent. Thyroid state normal.
	Kastin et al.	5	Four showed diminished responses.
1974	Coppen et al.	16	Four showed no response. Thyroid state normal.
	Chazot et al.	30	Fifteen showed diminished responses.
	Ehrensing et al.	8	Three showed diminished responses.
	Hutton	1	Baseline TSH as well as TSH response diminished.
	Takahasi et al.	36	Twelve showed diminished responses.
1975	van den Burg et al.	10	Mean TSH response diminished. Thyroid state normal.
	Kirkegaard et al.	15	Mean response diminished in depression as compared to recovery; diminished response related to early relapse.
	Widerlov and Sjostrom	10	Baseline TSH as well as TSH responses lower than in hospitalized, nondepressed controls.
	Maeda et al.	13	Mean response diminished as compared to controls.
1976	Pecknold et al.	6	Diminished in all patients. All patients euthyroid.
1977	Loosen et al.	23	Six showed diminished responses. No correlation

TABLE V (continued)

Reference	Year	N	Findings
			with age, severity of illness, clinical subtypes, or clinical remission.
Gold et al.		23	TSH responses lower in unipolar than in bipolar patients or controls. Negative correlation of CSF-5HIAA and baseline TSH.
Gregoire et al		19	TSH response to TRH diminished in depression, normalized after clinical remission.
Vogel et al.		15	Baseline TSH as well as response to TRH diminished.
Loosen et al.	1978	7	TSH blunting related to serum cortisol elevation.
Kirkegaard et al.		74	Mean TSH response diminished in manic depressive disease; normal in neurotic and reactive depression.

Depression - Negative Findings

Reference	Year	N	Findings
Shopsin et al.	1973	2	Responses normal.
Dimitrikoudi et al.	1974	2	Responses normal.
van den Burg et al.	1976	10	Responses normal. TRH infused during 4 hr period, possibly masking blunting.

Mania - Positive Finding

Reference	Year	N	Findings
Takahashi et al.	1974	8	TSH response somewhat diminished.
Kirkegaard et al.	1978	14	Tendency toward diminished response.

only on Factor I of the Hamilton Rating Scale for Depression (172), which is concerned mainly with motor retardation and depressed mood. Mean scores for the three treatment groups were significantly different at only one time period, three hours after injection. At later times, differences between treatment groups were slight with all groups showing a tendency to improve rapidly.

Huey et al. (122) injected TRH, 0.5 mg i.v., in three subjects in a state of predelirium tremens. They found no reliable beneficial effects. Two patients in milder stages of withdrawal showed a trend toward hormone effect revealed by improvement in sense of well-being and increased relaxation.

b. Endocrine Effects

TRH was injected in 12 chronic alcoholic men in AWS and in 10 alcoholic men after all symptoms of withdrawal had shown complete remission (PWS) (166, 168, 172). In AWS, 6 of 12 patients showed a blunted response of TSH to TRH challenge. To evaluate possible changes in individual TSH responses during the course of the disease, three of these six men with TSH blunting were retested in post-withdrawal syndrome (PWS). In two men the TSH response remained blunted while in one it normalized, suggesting that TSH blunting observed in AWS may or may not be corrected upon recovery. In addition, findings in AWS suggested thyroid activation and increased central dopaminergic activity as evidenced by elevated baseline GH, low baseline PRL, and a blunted TSH response to TRH. The former two abnormalities had normalized in PWS. However, a blunted TSH response was still seen in three of ten patients in PWS. None of these patients had received TRH in AWS. In contrast to patients with primary depression, in alcoholic men the TSH response was not related to serum cortisol levels. There was no significant correlation between basal cortisol and TSH response in either AWS or PWS.

Patients in AWS were classified as responders or as nonresponders in regard to their TSH responses. As mentioned above, six patients had shown a blunted response while six patients showed a normal response. Serum cortisol and thyroid hormone values did not differ between the two groups. However, TSH nonresponders showed significantly more behavioral improvement after TRH injection.

The data summarized above indicate that some depressed and some alcoholic patients share a deviant endocrine finding—a blunted TSH response to TRH. In both conditions the fault was observed in the acute state of the disease and, less often after symptoms had remitted. Thus it is possible that TSH blunting represents a common biological feature of both conditions which might parallel the genetic relationship between alcoholism in men and early onset unipolar depression in women suggested by Winokur et al. (301). Studies of family members of alcoholics and of alcoholics abstinent for an extended time are needed to clarify this possibility.

Previous studies of thyroid function in alcoholism have been addressed to patients in the chronic state rather than in the AWS. These data have been reviewed elsewhere (172, 261). In two studies which employed TRH in normal subjects given alcohol the TSH baseline was found unchanged, and after administration of TRH, the TSH and PRL peak responses were found to be normal (157, 302). However, about ten hours after the cessation of alcohol the PRL response to TRH was blunted (302). Unfortunately, the TSH response to TRH has not been reported in normals during alcohol withdrawal.

(3) Schizophrenia

a. *Behavioral Effects*

We described beneficial effects of TRH in four schizophrenic patients in a preliminary study (297). We have studied ten more patients in a double-blind trial in which i.v. nicotinic acid was used as an active placebo to mimic the occasional side effects of the peptide. TRH, 0.5 mg i.v., produced beneficial effects in patients in whom social withdrawal, anhedonia, and abulia were egregious symptoms. The duration of improvement was variable but averaged about ten days. TRH seemed to aggravate the mental state of a small subgroup of paranoid patients (unpublished observations).

Most authors have reported that TRH does exert behavioral effects in schizophrenia, though the effects are not always beneficial. In only three studies involving 25 patients has TRH been reported to be inactive. Drayson (70) reported the results of giving repeated injections of TRH, 0.2 mg, to three patients with "cyclical psychosis." None of his patients showed significant change. Clark et al. (44) performed a double-blind, placebo-controlled, crossover study of oral TRH, 300 mg per day, over three weeks. The 12 schizophrenic patients studied demonstrated no systematic behavioral changes. Lindstrom and his colleagues (159) studied ten chronic schizophrenic patients in a double-blind crossover design employing TRH, 0.6 mg i.v., on four consecutive days. The results of this study were substantially negative.

Three studies involving 212 schizophrenics have revealed beneficial effects. Inanaga et al. (125) administered oral TRH, 4 mg per day, in an open study of 62 chronic schizophrenic patients who concomitantly took standard neuroleptics. Reduced spontaneity, abulia, apathy, and social withdrawal were prominent symptoms. In about 75% of the patients a favorable response was observed within two weeks. The same investigators later treated 143 similar patients with oral TRH, 4 mg per day for 14 days, or with placebo, in a double-blind procedure (126). TRH was significantly more effective in producing overall improvement, especially in enhancing motivation and social contact. In a preliminary trial Campbell et al. (34) reported that TRH, 0.4 mg i.v., produced favorable behavioral changes in eight of ten autistic schizophrenic children.

Two studies involving 12 patients have reported unfavorable behavioral effects after TRH injection. Bigelow et al. (19) found slight worsening of depression in two of three treatment-resistant schizophrenics. Davis et al. (54) gave nine schizophrenic men TRH, 300 mg orally per day for 14 days, in an open trial. Seven patients worsened, an event especially marked in paranoid patients. One withdrawn schizophrenic showed clear improvement.

Although the results outlined above do not allow definitive conclusions, it can be suggested that chronic schizophrenic patients tend to benefit from TRH if they are not paranoid and especially if they prominently display symptoms of social withdrawal, abulia, and anhedonia. Paranoid patients may be worsened by administration of the peptide, and the differential effect may be another distinction between paranoid schizophrenics and nonparanoid schizophrenics (275). To the extent that TRH may have pro-dopaminergic activity (101), this notion weakens the relevance of the dopamine hypothesis (256) for nonparanoid schizophrenics.

b. Endocrine Effects

We found no TSH blunting in our schizophrenic patients (174), and this finding agreed with an earlier report (169). In contrast to depressed patients, schizophrenic patients showed a strong tendency toward a positive correlation between serum cortisol and TRH-induced TSH response (173, 174). In a recent preliminary study, Campbell et al. (34) reported deviant responses of TSH to

Psychotropic Drug Research

TRH in children with childhood schizophrenia with autistic features. Interestingly, children with the most deviant biological responses demonstrated the most marked behavioral changes after TRH injection.

(4) Other Disorders

a. Behavioral Effects

In male sexual impotence Benkert (14) found oral TRH no more effective than placebo in a double-blind, crossover study of 12 patients.

Several investigators have assessed the action of TRH in Parkinson's disease. Chase et al. (42) found that the hormone did not produce significant changes in neurological symptoms. However, their patients reported an increased sense of well-being and optimism. Lakke et al. (153) also found that the symptoms of Parkinson's disease were unaltered by TRH, though the hormone reduced depression scores. McCaul and his colleagues (183) found that two of three Parkinsonian patients taking L-dopa, when given TRH, experienced a "dramatic improvement in well-being, including enhanced clarity of thought." Neurologic symptoms were essentially unchanged.

Tiwary et al. (273) reported the results of a double-blind, crossover study of two hyperactive children. Both patients had responded poorly to methylphenidate administration. For two days after injection of TRH, 0.2 mg, most aspects of their behavior were notably improved.

b. Endocrine Effects

We are ignorant of studies of endocrine effects of TRH administration in male sexual impotence, Parkinson's disease, or hyperkinetic syndrome of children.

(5) Normal Subjects

a. Behavioral Effects

We performed a double-blind, crossover trial of TRH, 0.5 mg i.v., compared to saline, in ten normal women (298). Mental changes after saline were slight. After TRH, subjects showed significant relaxation, mild euphoria and increased energy. These changes were not related to frequency of side effects. We performed a similar study in 20 additional women and obtained similar results (Prange et al., unpublished data). Betts et al. (17) have confirmed these findings.

b. Endocrine Effects

In normals TRH causes the release of TSH and PRL, GH release being limited to pathological conditions (245). Peak TSH response is proportional to the dose of TRH over a broad range (6, 109, 254). Some authors (207, 294), but not all (109, 254, 255, 274), have reported that TSH responses are greater in women than in men. In a similar way, it has been reported that TSH response diminishes with age in men but not in women (294). Anderson et al. (6) suggested that a few normals, perhaps 5%, show no TSH response after TRH stimulation. We have not seen this phenomenon, however, in a series of more than 60 normals. Our subjects have shown a TSH response (rise above baseline) of 5 μU or more after 0.5 mg TRH i.v. In patients we have not counted a response as blunted unless it was less than this value.

B. Luteinizing Hormone Releasing Hormone (LHRH)

LHRH is a decapeptide (pGlu-His-Trp-Ser-Tyr-Gly-Leu-Arg-Pro-Gly-NH$_2$) characterized in the laboratories of Guillemin (106) and Schally (246). It causes the release of the two anterior pituitary gonadotropins, luteinizing hormone (LH) and follicle stimulating hormone (FSH). As noted, the most striking behavioral effect of LHRH in animals is induction of lordosis behavior in female rats (191, 192).

(1) Affective Disorders

a. Behavioral Effects

Benkert (14) gave LHRH (or TRH) or saline, each on one occasion, to a small group of depressed patients. Both hormones were somewhat more effective than saline, though the effect of neither was statistically superior to that of saline.

b. Endocrine Effects

Very little is known of possible alterations in the hypothalamic-pituitary-gonadal (HPG) axis in depressed patients. The lack of

135

endocrine studies in this area is striking (226), especially if one considers that disturbances in sexual behavior are prominent symptoms in depression.

In a recent report by Ettigi and Brown (82) LHRH was injected in a group of depressed patients. The authors reported a significantly increased LH response to LHRH in men with secondary depression if compared to men with primary unipolar depression.

(2) Alcoholism

a. Behavioral Effects

No studies have been addressed to the possible behavioral effects of LHRH in alcoholism.

b. Endocrine Effects

There is abundant evidence for disturbances in the HPG axis in alcoholic patients. Alcoholic men often show hyperestrogenization and hypoandrogenization, possibly related to liver damage (185, 272). Two studies have employed LHRH in normal subjects given alcohol (157, 302). In both studies the LH response to LHRH did not change after drinking was started.

(3) Schizophrenia

a. Behavioral Effects

No studies have been addressed to the possible behavioral effects of LHRH in schizophrenia.

b. Endocrine Effects

Brambilla et al. (29) performed LHRH injections in chronic schizophrenic patients. They noted increases in both TSH and LH which were greater than those of control subjects.

(4) Male Sexual Impotence

a. Behavioral Effects

Three groups have given LHRH, all by different routes, to impotent men with or without evidence of endocrine disorder, and quite variable results have been obtained (228). Mortimer et al. (190) suggested that LHRH may exert a behavioral effect independent of its endocrine effects in selected patients: "In six of the seven adult patients there was an early increase in potency, 7 to 14 days after starting therapy, which was maintained despite circulating 17-β-hydroxyandrogen levels well below the lower limit of the normal male range."

b. Endocrine Effects

Delilala et al. (55) injected LHRH in men with psychogenic impotence and did not find reliable differences of LH and TSH responses if compared to responses evoked in normal controls.

(5) Other Disorders

a. Behavioral Effects

Possible behavioral effects of LHRH have not been studied in anorexia nervosa or in Huntington's chorea.

b. Endocrine Effects

There is evidence for disturbances in the HPG axis in patients with anorexia nervosa. Diminished basal LH levels and a disturbed circadian pattern of LH secretion have been reported. LH and LH reactivity to LHRH seem to relate to the patient's weight loss and body fat though data on this point are still conflicting (for reviews see 111, 131, 140).

A recent study has demonstrated a marked increase in the concentration of immunoreactive LHRH in the median eminence of women who have suffered from Huntington's chorea (20). The significance of this finding is not well understood.

(6) Normal Subjects

a. Behavioral Effects

McAdoo et al. (182) gave LHRH to normal males and found "increase in alertness, decrease in anxiety and fatigue, and an increased speed of performance on automatized motor tasks . . ." These authors also noted a significant increase in self-reported sexual arousal after LHRH administration. La Ferla et al. (152)

Psychotropic Drug Research

showed that the viewing of an erotic film caused enhanced LH secretion. After LHRH injection the magnitude of LH response was found to be positively correlated with the subjective evaluation of sexual arousal. These data, taken together, indicate that LHRH may be involved in sexual arousal in man.

b. Endocrine Effects

LHRH causes the anterior pituitary gland to release LH and FSH in a dose-related fashion (106, 246).

C. Melanocyte Stimulating Hormone Release Inhibiting Factor (MIF-I)

MIF-I is Pro-Leu-Gly-NH$_2$; it inhibits release by the anterior pituitary gland of melanocyte stimulating hormone (MSH) (191). It is of interest to note that Pro-Leu-Gly-NH$_2$ also occurs as the side chain of the oxytocin molecule (197).

(1) Affective Disorders

a. Behavioral Effects

In a double-blind study Ehrensing and Kastin (74) treated 18 depressed women. Six received MIF-I, 60 mg per day p.o.; six received 150 mg; six received placebo capsules. The authors reported a marked prompt improvement from the lower doses of the tripeptide. In a second double-blind, placebo-controlled study the same authors treated 24 patients who had either bipolar or unipolar depression (76). For six days patients received MIF-I orally, 75 or 750 mg per day, or placebo. As in their first study, these workers found that only the smaller dose of the tripeptide produced a significant antidepressant effect.

MIF-I has not been given to manic patients.

b. Endocrine Effects

The endocrine effects of MIF-I administration have not been studied in patients with affective disorders.

(2) Parkinson's Disease

a. Behavioral Effects

While both TRH and MIF-I potentiate the behavioral effects of L-dopa in mice (214, 215, 216), MIF-I is clearly more potent (120).

Peptides in Mental Disorders

This suggests that MIF-I might exert a greater benefit than TRH in Parkinson's disease, and this appears to be the case. All trials of MIF-I in Parkinson's disease have produced positive results (12, 135). Large doses of MIF-I have been used, a tactic that is permitted by the fact that the pituitary secretions affected by MIF-I, unlike those affected by, say, TRH, lack a discrete target organ. MIF-I, of course, inhibits the release of MSH. This hormone has been reported to be elevated in patients with Parkinson's disease, and its administration exacerbates Parkinsonian symptoms (139). Whether the benefits of MIF-I in Parkinson's disease are related to dopamine activation or to MSH inhibition is uncertain.

In an open study of ten patients with Parkinson's disease, Gerstenbrand and his co-workers (91) injected MIF-I, 400 mg i.v. per day for ten days. In addition to beneficial effects on neurologic symptoms, an antidepressant effect of MIF-I was observed. Seven patients were found to be depressed before treatment; after treatment four patients showed remission from depression, one patient showed symptoms of hypermania, and two patients were still depressed.

b. Endocrine Effects

The endocrine effects of MIF-I administration have not been studied in Parkinson's disease.

D. Somatotropin Release Inhibiting Factor (SRIF, somatostatin)

SRIF is a tetradecapeptide (H-Ala-Gly-Cys-Lys-Asn-Phe-Phe-Trp-Lys-Thr-Phe-Thr-Ser-Lys-OH) (30). A disulfide bond connects the two cysteine residues. It inhibits the release of GH (30, 251). In the periphery it has a variety of effects, including complicated effects on insulin (73) and glucose metabolism (90).

(1) Parkinson's Disease

a. Behavioral Effects

Cotzias et al. (50) injected SRIF, 2 mg i.v., in three patients with Parkinson's disease undergoing L-dopa therapy. SRIF infusion "produced a diminution of the antiparkinson, and more so, of the dyskinetic effects of L-dopa." Thus SRIF tended to offset both the therapeutic and the unwanted effects of L-dopa.

b. Endocrine Effects

In the study mentioned above SRIF infusion in Parkinson's dis-

Psychotropic Drug Research

ease resulted in a diminution of serum GH and L-dopa levels.

III. ANTERIOR PITUITARY HORMONES

A. Adrenocorticotropin (ACTH) and Related Peptides

Of all the anterior pituitary hormones, the corticotropin-related peptides have received the most attention as behaviorally active substances and we have reviewed both the animal and clinical data in detail (202, 203, 228).

de Wied and his collaborators (58, 60, 62, 64-66) have conclusively demonstrated that the release of ACTH results in important effects on the acquisition and maintenance of behavioral processes. ACTH is a 39-membered amino acid chain (51). It bears certain resemblances to β-lipotropin, fragments of which contain the amino acid sequences of α, β, and γ-endorphin as well as methionine-enkephalin but not leucine-enkephalin (Figure 1). The first 13 amino acids of ACTH occur in the same sequence as the 13 amino acids that comprise the molecule of α-MSH. Thus $ACTH_{1-13}$ and α-MSH possess the identical amino sequence though the latter contains a 1-acetyl and a 13-terminal NH_2.

Attention was focused on corticotropin-related peptides when it became clear that treatment with these compounds restored certain behavioral deficits present in hypophysectomized animals (60, 62, 66). The fact that corticosteroids were ineffective in restoring such deficits suggested that the ACTH effect was not due to adrenal activation. Further study showed that fragments of the ACTH molecule virtually devoid of corticotropin activity (α-MSH, $ACTH_{4-10}$, $ACTH_{4-7}$, etc.) are active in restoring the learning deficits (in both active and passive avoidance behavior) of hypophysectomized animals (66). Since these effects are also observed after CNS administration of ACTH and related fragments, the available data taken together indicate that ACTH and related peptides exert their effects directly on the CNS and certainly are not mediated by the adrenal cortex.

de Wied and his collaborators have also examined the effects of ACTH and its analogs in intact animals. Although acquisition of active avoidance behavior appeared to be unaffected, extinction of these responses was markedly delayed by corticotropin-related peptides. ACTH and related peptides delayed extinction of conditioned behavior whether motivated by hunger, fear, or taste aversion (60, 62, 64-66). ACTH and its analogs have been reported to affect

140

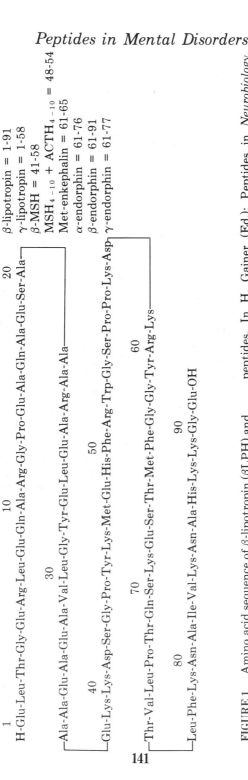

FIGURE 1 Amino acid sequence of β-lipotropin (βLPH) and peptides contained within the β-LPH molecule. Adapted from de Wied, D., and Gispen, W.H.: Behavioral effects of peptides. In H. Gainer (Ed.): Peptides in *Neurobiology*, Plenum Press, New York, 1977, with permission.

many other behaviors (27, 209, 235, 248). For example, Kastin et al. (137) propose that $ACTH_{1-13}$ and related peptides facilitate the attentive ability or motivation of a rat.

Structure-activity studies with ACTH congeners have provided interesting data on the molecular requirements for behavioral activity. Comparisons have been made in potency of substances in inhibiting the extinction of pole-jumping avoidance behavior (62, 65). In this paradigm a light is turned on five seconds before a footshock is applied. The rat must jump on a pole to avoid the shock. After the rat learns avoidance, the light is still presented though the shock is no longer delivered. For a time rats continue to jump on the pole, but finally they do not, that is, they show extinction. Active compounds, given subcutaneously, either delay or facilitate extinction. The tetrapeptide $ACTH_{4-7}$ is the smallest fragment that possesses behavioral activity, and it delays extinction. It is interesting to note that in this latter paradigm, LHRH is equipotent with $ACTH_{4-10}$ and TRH is one-third as active (65).

Our group (21, 24) found that several behaviorally active ACTH fragments and analogs (e.g., $ACTH_{4-7NH_2}$) significantly antagonized pentobarbital-induced narcosis and hypothermia.

In the paragraphs below we shall outline the behavioral effects of ACTH and related peptides in humans. Generally when behavioral effects have been studied, endocrine effects have been neglected. (Indeed, some behaviorally active molecules are largely devoid of endocrine effects.) There is, of course, an extensive literature pertaining to the status of the adrenal axis in mental disorders. The affective disorders, particularly depression, have been most extensively studied and the administration of ACTH has played a role in this field. A strong consensus exists that in a large minority of depressed patients there is central disinhibition of the pituitary-adrenal axis (41, 226).

(1) Schizophrenia

Endroczi (80) has summarized the work conducted by his group on the effects of $ACTH_{1-10}$ "in extreme depressive states (schizophrenic patients) daily treatment with 3-6 mg of the ACTH fragment resulted in elimination of the depressive state, increase in communication, and mood elevation. These effects were observed within 5-7 days."

(2) Hyperkinetic Syndrome of Children

Rapoport et al. (232) evaluated the effects of $ACTH_{4-10}$ treatment in hyperactive, learning-disabled children. Measures of visual and auditory memory, new learning, impulsivity, attention, perceptual motor skills, and anxiety were analyzed after 30 mg (i.m.) of the peptide. No significant effects were observed.

Sandman and his colleagues (241) have reported that in a double-blind study $ACTH_{4-10}$ dramatically improved the performance of mentally retarded subjects in visual discrimination and memory tests. In addition van Riezen et al. (283) have cited the unpublished work of Wagenaar, who has found that $ACTH_{4-10}$ treatment one week *post training* in normal volunteers significantly enhanced retrieval.

(3) Convulsive Disorders

Klein (146) has summarized studies conducted by his group and others on the effects of ACTH and corticosteroids in epileptiform disorders. Treatment with these agents frequently results in dramatic improvements (decreased seizures and normalization of the EEG pattern) in patients suffering from convulsive disorders. Whether the ACTH effects observed in these studies are due to direct CNS actions of this peptide or mediated via the pituitary-adrenal axis is undetermined.

(4) Other Disorders

Strand and her colleagues (262) have studied the effects of ACTH fragments on muscle action potentials in animals and man. In two patients, one with myasthenia gravis and another with progressive spinal muscular atrophy, the peptide prevented the pathological decline in amplitude in a series of evoked muscle action potentials.

Cotzias et al. (49) reported that large doses of MSH aggravated Parkinson's disease.

Recently Henderson et al. (114) have analyzed data derived from a multicenter study of ACTH in multiple sclerosis; the peptide produced a significant improvement in neurological function.

(5) Normal Subjects

Endroczi and co-workers (79) studied the effects of ACTH and ACTH fragments on stimulus-induced EEG synchrony in 16 human subjects. The administration of 50 units of $ACTH_{1-10}$ or $ACTH_{1-24}$ was followed by suppression of the number of synchronized EEG responses and the effect lasted at least two days.

143

Higher doses led to a marked suppression of the stimulus-induced EEG synchronization. $ACTH_{11-24}$ was ineffective in this regard. The EEG patterns returned to normal about five days after treatment.

Kastin and his co-workers have reported extensively on the effects of ACTH, α-MSH, and related peptides on behavioral and electrographic measures in man, and these data have recently been reviewed (138). In an early study (134) infusion of 10 mg of α-MSH caused marked increases in the averaged somatosensory cortical evoked response during relaxation. This effect was even greater during attention. Although verbal retention was unaltered, α-MSH administration was associated with increased visual retention. There was also a tendency toward a slowing of the EEG frequency. The administration of α-MSH_{4-10} (structurally identical to $ACTH_{4-10}$) (see Figure 1) to 20 normal young men revealed results similar to those obtained with α-MSH. Visual discrimination and retention, both of which can be considered sensitive indicators of the state of attention of the subject were significantly improved. Spatial perception was also improved. This same group has studied the effects of injection of either $ACTH_{1-24}$ or $ACTH_{4-10}$ (10 mg as a bolus) on a battery of bioelectric and behavioral measures of attention, memory, and anxiety in man during a dysjunctive reactive time paradigm (187). Although $ACTH_{1-24}$ had no marked effects on any of the measures examined, $ACTH_{4-10}$ improved visual memory, decreased anxiety, reinstated a previously habituated alpha-blocking response in the occipital EEG, and influenced the occipital EEG in a manner interpreted as increased attention. Furthermore, these investigators observed EEG responses similar to those obtained by Endroczi, as cited above. In contrast, Sannita et al. (243) found that the i.v. administration of $ACTH_{4-10}$ (60 mg) produced no statistically significant changes in the EEG or behavior of 12 normal male volunteers. In only one test (digital span test) did the subjects show a decrease in the number of errors.

Gaillard and Sanders (89) have reported that the s.c. injection of 30 mg $ACTH_{4-10}$ to 18 human subjects resulted in a significant improvement in reaction time during the experimental session in a self-paced reaction task, as well as a reduction in the number of errors made. The effect was short-lived; it disappeared when measured in a retest administered 30 minutes after the experiment. The authors hypothesized that this peptide suppresses the decrease in motivation normally associated with continuous performance tasks. Subjective ratings were in agreement with this interpretation.

Peptides in Mental Disorders

In a recent double-blind study Sandman et al. (242) have reported that infusion of 11 normal male volunteers (age 21-25) with $ACTH_{4-10}$ (15 mg over a two hour period) produced *impaired* performance in a detection task, but enhanced performance in a discrimination task. They interpret their results to indicate that $ACTH_{4-10}$ uniquely affects attentional processes. Miller et al. (188) have recently reported that administration of 30 mg $ACTH_{4-10}$ (s.c.) exerts no significant effect on any parameter of acquisition or extinction of an active conditioned avoidance response in human volunteers.

B. Thyroid Stimulating Hormone (TSH)

As mentioned above ACTH appears to be localized in brain as well as in anterior pituitary. Recently Moldow and Yalow (189) have reported that TSH occurs in the hypothalamus as well as the anterior pituitary of man and is even more widely distributed in rat brain. The pituitary does, however, appear to be the only site of synthesis.

(1) Affective Disorders

a. Behavioral Effects

We performed a double-blind, placebo-controlled study to discern whether bovine TSH, 10 IU administered i.m., would accelerate the antidepressant action of imipramine in depressed women (219). Patients who received imipramine plus the hormone improved more rapidly than those who received imipramine plus saline injection. In this experiment TSH may have exerted an antidepressant effect independent of the endocrine effects. However, a sufficient explanation for the finding is that imipramine potentiation was the consequence of enhanced thyroid hormone secretion prompted by TSH. This interpretation is consistent with the findings of previous studies in which it was shown that oral administration of L-triiodothyronine also accelerates the therapeutic action of imipramine in depressed women (218, 296).

b. Endocrine Effects

In the study described above the endocrine responses of depressed women were almost identical to those reported in normal women. Total serum thyroxine doubled within 24 hours of TSH injection.

Psychotropic Drug Research

Thus, thyroidal reserve appears to be normal in depressed patients.

Weeke and Weeke (293) have shown that in severe endogenous depression there is loss of diurnal rhythmicity of TSH, due mainly to loss of nocturnal elevation of levels.

C. Growth Hormone (GH)

GH has been found to reduce the incidence of restraint-induced gastric erosion in rats (285). Recently the same group of investigators (299) have shown that human GH tends to heal stress ulcers in patients with neoplasms. Direct mucosal effects of the hormone provide a sufficient explanation for the observation. Nevertheless, it would be premature to exclude possible CNS effects as playing a role, especially since stress ulcer can occur in a variety of conditions, including cerebral lesions.

In man GH appears to prolong the half-life of amobarbital, presumably through an action on hepatic microsomal systems (233).

IV. POSTERIOR PITUITARY HORMONES

A. Vasopressin (VP)

The posterior lobe of the pituitary gland secretes two peptides, vasopressin (VP) and oxytocin (OXT), both of which are elaborated in brain. VP, synthesized mostly in the supraoptic nucleus, conserves body water by reducing water excretion by the kidney and increases vascular smooth muscle tone (145). VP is also called antidiuretic hormone (ADH). OXT, synthesized largely in the paraventricular nucleus, facilitates milk ejection (145). It is commonly used as a therapeutic agent to produce uterine contraction.

de Wied and his colleagues have evaluated the role of VP and related substances in learning and memory processes (59, 63, 64, 66). Although removal of the posterior and intermediate lobes in rats does not change the rate of *acquisition* of conditioned avoidance behavior, it results in changes in the rate of *extinction*. Rats lacking the neurohypophysis do not show the resistance to extinction observed in intact control animals, that is, they "forget" quicker. They simply are unable to maintain a learned response unless punishment is applied. Early studies showed that a crude posterior pituitary extract (pitressin) normalizes this deficit in hypophysectomized animals and increases resistance to extinction of a shuttlebox avoidance response. The remarkable finding in

146

these experiments was the fact that the behavioral effects of pitressin injection lasted for weeks after treatment had been discontinued. VP was found to be the active principle in pitressin injection since equimolar injections of OXT were without effect (59).

Evidence that the behavioral effects of VP are independent of its classical endocrine actions come from studies with analogs of the hormone. Desglycinamidelysine-8-vasopressin, an endogenous hog pituitary peptide that has virtually no pressor or antidiuretic activity, is extremely effective in normalizing the behavioral deficits characteristic of posterior-lobectomized rats (61,63,236).

A series of recent reports suggest that the behavioral actions of VP are physiologic [see de Wied and Gispen (66) for review]. The first bit of evidence comes from studies comparing the effectiveness of intracerebroventricular (i.c.v.) vs peripheral administration of the peptide. The i.c.v. injection of VP affects extinction of the pole-jumping avoidance response at doses 200-fold less than needed for systemic administration (66). Another approach has been the use of specific antisera to VP, which presumably inactivates endogenous VP. The i.c.v. administration of VP (but not growth hormone or OXT) antiserum after a learning trial leads to a deficit in passive avoidance retention (284). The peripheral injection of large quantities of VP antiserum (sufficient to neutralize circulating plasma VP) has no such effect, providing further evidence for a brain locus of action of VP. Lesion and microinjection data indicate that midbrain limbic structures (septum and dorsal hippocampus) mediate the behavioral effects of VP analogs (66). In recent years de Wied's group (284) has utilized the Brattleboro strain of rats, which lack the ability to synthesize VP and consequently have hereditary diabetes insipidis. These animals have marked memory deficits that can readily be reversed by the s.c. injection of μg of desglycinamide-lysine-8-vasopressin. The abnormal EEG patterns characteristic of Brattleboro rats can also be normalized by treatment with VP analogs (66).

Further evidence for a role of VP in memory processes comes from recent studies that have shown that this neurohypophysial hormone and related analogs prevent puromycin-induced amnesia in mice (291) and CO_2-induced and electroshock-induced amnesia in the rat (235). This array of results has led to a hypothesis of the role of VP in behavioral homeostasis. It is part of a larger hypothesis that postulates that neuropeptides released from the pituitary are involved in the formation and maintenance of new behavioral patterns. Unlike the behavioral effects of corticotropin-

Psychotropic Drug Research

related peptides, which are short-lived, the effects of VP and VP analogs are long-lived. This distinction has been observed in both hypophysectomized and intact animals. The VP effect may involve consolidation of memory processes (66).

To the best of our knowledge pitressin is the only posterior pituitary hormone for which a behavioral claim is made in humans. Pitressin is a purified extract of posterior pituitary glands in which VP has been retained and OXT excluded. More than 20 years ago Forizs and his colleagues used repeated injections of this substance to treat chronic schizophrenic patients. Guided by the belief that schizophrenia and epilepsy are incompatible disorders, they proposed shifting water metabolism toward a pattern more characteristic of patients with epilepsy. In a series of studies, uncontrolled but involving many patients, the treatment showed early promise (85). It was abandoned with the advent of modern neuroleptic drugs (L. Forizs, personal communication, 1975). We are not aware of recent studies on behavioral effects of VP in man. It should be noted, however, that Gold et al. (96) have summarized the evidence that suggests a possible role of VP in affective disorders.

V. OPIATE RELATED SUBSTANCES

Of all the advances in neuroscience in the past decade, few have received as much attention as the finding that the brain and pituitary contain peptide substances that possess analgesic activity and interact with opiate receptors in the brain and periphery. We have reviewed the early findings in this field prior to chemical characterization of the endogenous opiate ligands (228); others have written more recent and comprehensive reviews (48, 98, 286).

The formulas of leu- and met-enkephalin, the endorphins and their relation to ACTH and β-lipotropin (β-LPH) are illustrated in Figure 1. In general, the enkephalins are heterogenously distributed in the CNS of various laboratory animals whereas the endorphins and β-LPH are found mainly in the pituitary gland. However, β-endorphins and β-LPH also appear to exist in the brain and enkephalin-like activity has been reported in the pituitary (2,25). The CNS distribution of opiate-like substances, like other aspects of this field, is rife with controversy. For example, Liotta et al. (160) have been unable to find β-endorphin in human pituitary. Blume et al. (26) have discovered an endogenous opiate-like substance that is not a peptide.

It is clear that a family of endogenous opiate-like peptides exist

148

and more members may await discovery. Certainly other peptides appear to exert analgesic effects: for example, neurotensin (NT) (45,204) and substance P (87). The effects of these peptides, unlike those of the endorphins and enkephalins, are not naloxone-reversible. In fact, some of the effects of the endorphins and enkephalins are not naloxone-reversible. These findings reveal the complex nature of the brain's analgesic systems and perhaps this intricacy will, as Goldstein and Hansteen (99) have suggested, "have value in damping the wildfire of speculations that have recently plagued both the scientific and popular media."

Terenius and Wahlstrom (271) have noted three strategies that have been employed to evaluate the functional role of opiate-like peptides in man: (1) observations in humans treated with opiate-like peptides; (2) administration to humans of opiate antagonists (e.g. naloxone and naltrexone), which presumably block the effects of endogenous opiate-like peptides, and subsequent evaluation of induced changes in behavior, physiology, etc. and; (3) measurement of opiate-like peptides in body fluids and tissues of patients with neurological and psychiatric disorders. We shall briefly review the salient findings derived from each of these strategies.

A. Depression and Schizophrenia

In an uncontrolled study performed by Kline et al. (147) six patients (three depressed, three schizophrenic) received various doses of β-endorphin (1.5-8 mg i.v.). All three schizophrenic patients rapidly improved as regards cognitive impairment and two of the depressed patients exhibited improvement in mood. On second injection larger doses of β-endorphin were administered, but no objective or subjective changes were noted.

de Wied and his colleagues (67,287) have presented data that Des-Tyr^1-γ-endorphin possesses neuroleptic activity as measured in effects on extinction of a pole-jumping avoidance task, and based on this they have administered the peptide to six schizophrenic patients. All showed transient improvement (diminished frequency of hallucinations and other psychotic symptoms), though neuropeptide treatment had to be withdrawn from three patients because of apparent exacerbation of psychotic symptomatology. From these data de Wied and Van Ree (68) have suggested first that Des-Tyr^1-γ-endorphin is an endogenous neuroleptic and furthermore that a reduced availability of this peptide may well be an etiological factor in the pathogenesis of schizophrenia.

149

Psychotropic Drug Research

(1) Pain States

Catlin et al. (41) administered human β-endorphin (6-440 μg/kg i.v.) to three patients with cancer pain and two patients undergoing methadone withdrawal. Two of the cancer patients reported significant pain relief though one of these also responded to injection of saline. Both methadone-dependent subjects reported a complete relief of narcotic abstinence symptoms after β-endorphin administration 440 μg/kg i.v.). The effects of the peptide were subjectively judged as being different from morphine by one of these patients. Hosobuchi and Li (120) administered β-endorphin (100, 200, or 400 μg) ICV in a double-blind study to three patients suffering from untractable pain. Substantial pain relief was produced as measured with a thermal dolorometer and the effect lasted 4-8 hours. These effects were naloxone-reversible.

(2) Normal Subjects

Von Graffenreid et al. (290) evaluated the effects of 0.1-1.2 mg i.v. of a potent synthetic analog of met-enkephalin (FK-33-824) in 40 male volunteers in a single-blind study. No changes in blood pressure, pulse rate, respiratory rate, body temperature, EKG profile, or standard clinical chemistry and hematological tests were observed. The most frequent effect reported was a "feeling of heaviness in all the muscles of the body often combined with a feeling of oppression on the chest or tightness in the throat." Other effects noted were a marked increase in bowel sounds and redness of the face. Well-known effects of morphine and morphinomimetics such as alterations in emotion and mental alertness were not observed. The enkephalin analog prompted the secretion of GH and PRL in a dose-dependent manner, and this confirmed observations made in animals (46). Of particular interest was the finding that these endocrine effects were not prevented by pretreatment with an opiate antagonist. The effects of this enkephalin analog on pituitary hormone secretion are apparently not a nonspecific stress response since plasma cortisol showed no significant change. An EEG profile was studied in 12 subjects and spectral analysis revealed slowing of α-waves, increase in electrical output in the α and β band, and a decrease in slow waves. These effects were also not reversed by nalorphine.

B. Effects of Opiate Antagonists

The interpretation of data concerning the effects of narcotic antagonists, such as naloxone, naltrexone, or nalorphine, is based on the assumption that such treatment antagonizes the activity of endogenous opiate-like substances. In this connection it is well to recall that opiate antagonists do not block all the effects of endogenous opiate-like substances when they are administered (290). Furthermore certain antagonists, notably nalorphine (72), have substantial agonist effects.

(1) Schizophrenia

Gunne et al. (107) found marked improvement in psychotic symptoms minutes after i.m. injection of 0.4 mg of naloxone. Several groups have been unable to confirm these findings (52,133,151, 289); however, in two recent studies naloxone was found to be superior to placebo. Watson et al. (292) found, in a double-blind cross-over study, that naloxone (0.4-1.2 mg) produced decreases in auditory hallucinations in some chronic schizophrenics. Herz et al. (116) reported that in a double-blind study of 20 patients who exhibited frequent hallucinations and delusions, naloxone (4 mg i.v.) produced a greater reduction in psychotic symptoms than did saline, though statistical analysis was not presented. Verebey et al. (286) has reviewed the data concerning naltrexone and schizophrenia; no salutary effects have been observed.

If the findings outlined immediately above and the data listed in the preceding section are taken as evidence, respectively, that both endorphins and naloxone exert antischizophrenic actions, one may wonder how an antagonist of a system and an agonist of the same system could exert similar effects. Indeed, this juxtaposition of findings may amount to a contradiction, but it need not. It now appears that there are several subgroups of schizophrenics (162), and perhaps different subgroups respond differentially to opiates and their blockers. A similar conundrum arises in connection with manipulations of dopamine, excess activity of which is considered by many to provide the biological substrate for schizophrenia (162). Dopamine receptor antagonists are acknowledged antipsychotic agents (162), apomorphine, a dopaminergic *agonist* has been reported to possess antischizophrenic properties as well (268).

(2) Pain States and Normal Subjects

On the whole, effects of naloxone have been difficult to demonstrate in untreated humans and animals (286), though the drug clearly antagonizes the majority of the effects of morphine, enkephalins, and endorphins. Thresholds to electrically-induced or ischemic pain is unaffected by naloxone administration. However, Levine et al. (158) have reported that following the extraction of impacted wisdom teeth, naloxone significantly increases reported pain intensity. Naloxone was found in a double-blind study to exert no significant effect on sexual arousal and orgasm in an adult male volunteer (99). It also reportedly does not alter hypnotic analgesia (97).

Davis et al. (53) administered 2 mg of naloxone to six sleeping young male volunteers. No sleep variables exhibited any significant change, and the authors suggested that endogenous opiate systems are not primarily involved in human sleep.

C. Measurement of Endorphins in Human CSF

This strategy assumes that deviation in levels of immunoreactive endorphins or enkephalins or in activity of CSF samples in an opiate receptor binding assay in different patient populations will reveal subgroups with endorphin-enkephalin hypo- or hyperactivity. Clearly, the meager endorphin and naloxone data cited above would predict both decreases (if schizophrenia is an endorphin-deficiency disease) and increases (if schizophrenia is naloxone-treatable) in endorphin levels in the brains of schizophrenics. Since all measurements have been performed on lumbar CSF samples, there is the additional problem of assuming that lumbar samples represent the functional activity of the CNS opiate systems involved in schizophrenia. Another important consideration is, of course, the specificity of the assays employed. The problems of specificity in radioimmunoassay (RIA) and radioreceptor assay of peptides has been discussed by Terenius and Wahlstrom (271) and by Youngblood et al. (303). Stringent analytical techniques must be utilized in addition to standard RIA procedures in order to determine the presence of potential nonspecific cross-reacting material. The radioreceptor assay simply measures material which occupies receptor sites. Neither procedure necessarily measures exclusively substances with biological activity.

(1) Depression

Terenius and Wahlstrom (271) have pioneered the research on measuring opiate-like activity in CSF from psychiatric and chronic pain patients. Two fractions (I & II) with opiate-like activity in the radioceptor assay and the RIA for met-enkephalin have been isolated from human CSF. They are thought not to represent any previously known endorphins. These workers found that control values from healthy volunteers fall within narrow limits whereas psychotic patients exhibited a large range of values. Patients with depression reportedly had higher levels of Fraction I and II endorphin. Terenius et al. (270) administered naloxone (0.4-0.8 mg tid) to five depressed patients, and though no mood change was evident, Fraction I levels of endorphin decreased (but not to control values) and CSF 5-hydroxy-indoleacetic acid levels, indicators of serotonin metabolism, increased in four of six trials. Mood deterioration occurred in two patients.

(2) Pain States and Normal Subjects

Akil and colleagues (3) have characterized an enkephalin-like substance in normal human CSF which resembles met-enkephalin in two chromatographic systems and the RIA for the pentapeptide. Its identity is not fully determined, but it clearly possesses activity in the radioreceptor assay. Patients with chronic pain had lower CSF levels of this opiate-like activity, but this difference did not achieve statistical significance. More recently, Akil et al. (1) have reported that electrical stimulation of periventricular brain sites in patients with intractable pain results in a significant diminution in their persistent pain. This analgesia was naloxone-reversible and associated with a significant rise in CSF enkephalin-like activity. Sjolund et al. (252) found that fraction I activity was low in chronic pain patients, and electro-acupuncture of the spinal cord increased this opiate activity in four patients (252).

Sicuteri et al. (250) utilized the assay system of Terenius and Wahlstrom (271) cited above and found the lowest endorphin levels in headache patients with pain whereas levels in patients without pain were 3- to 4-fold higher.

Sarne et al. (244) have reported on the presence in human CSF of an enkephalin-like substance which reacts with leu-enkephalin antibody. This opioid is larger than the enkephalins and considerably more stable.

(3) Other Disorders

A very high level of morphine-like factor activity has been seen in a single patient with the Guillain-Barre syndrome (250).

VI. OTHER PEPTIDES

A. Insulin

The earliest, best known, and most dramatic use of a polypeptide in clinical psychiatry is the administration of insulin to patients with psychiatric disorders. Shortly after its isolation in 1922 insulin was used to stimulate appetite in mental patients (13, 108, 230, 269). However, behavioral improvement discordant with nutritional improvement was sometimes noted (13,230). In 1928 Schmidt (247) performed the first systematic study of the effects of insulin on psychotic symptoms. Beneficial effects were noted, even when insulin administration was accompanied by carbohydrate administration to prevent hypoglycemia. This phenomenon—benefits from insulin if administered together with carbohydrates—has been widely confirmed (9,16,130,195,247,253) and received (237).

In 1935 Sakel (240) described "insulin shock treatment," which involved severe hypoglycemia and coma. Since then it has commonly been assumed that hypoglycemia plays an important, if not crucial, role in the therapeutic action of insulin in psychotic disorders. However, work from the preceding decade preserves the possibility that insulin, besides its many endocrine effects, may have direct effects on brain that in some patients result in improved behavior.

Insulin does appear to penetrate the blood-brain barrier (231), and recently, rat brain has been shown to contain insulin receptors (113). Rafaelsen and Mellerup (231) have listed the direct effects of insulin in animals, i.e., those effects that occur when hypoglycemia is avoided. Insulin, without producing hypoglycemia, may influence tryptophan metabolism in brain (266), though not all authors agree with this concept (175).

B. Glutathione

Glutathione, a tripeptide (γ-glutamyl-cysteinyl-glycine) plays an important role in oxidation-reduction systems of the cell. It is widely distributed in animal and plant cells and is found predominantly intracellularly. Its fundamental biological role and chemistry have been thoroughly reviewed (18,184).

Several enzymes related to carbohydrate and lipid metabolism depend on glutathione for their activity (184). When in the early 1950s Altschule and his co-workers (5,115) described a disorder of carbohydrate metabolism in patients with schizophrenic, manic-depressive, or involutional psychoses, the same workers (4) and others (10,11,71,181) investigated the role of glutathione in these disorders. However, data pertaining to glutathione serum levels in mentally ill patients are inconclusive. Both diminished (5,10,181) and normal (11,71,78) levels of the tripeptide have been reported. In an early study (7) glutathione (50 mg) was given to a heterogenous group of mentally ill patients whose diagnoses included neuroses, psychoses, and borderline states. In this study a uniformly beneficial affect was observed resulting "partly in reducing states of tension, anxiety, insomnia, and nervous irritability."

In 1957 Altschule et al. (4) injected glutathione, 0.5 gm/kg body weight, in five mentally ill patients. These investigators were mainly interested in the effect of glutathione on carbohydrate metabolism, but they assessed global clinical changes as well. One patient, diagnosed as "psychoneurotic, depressive reaction" did not show behavioral improvement. However, three patients diagnosed as "manic depressive psychosis, depressed phase," showed clinical improvement after tripeptide injection. In two of these patients a remission of depressive symptoms occurred, while one patient reported increased "feeling of relaxation." Moreover, one patient diagnosed as a paranoid schizophrenic and described as "vague, apathetic, withdrawn, and not communicating" improved clinically after 11 infusions of glutathione. "Two became sociable and showed interest in reading . . . (and were) . . . no longer mute. However, this improvement was maintained for less than a week after the last infusion." Since all patients showed changes in carbohydrate intermediate metabolism after glutathione injection it is difficult to assess whether a direct effect of glutathione accounted for the behavioral changes observed.

C. Threonyl–valyl–leucine

Gottlieb and Frohman (100) have purportedly indentified a serum α-2-globulin (MW 263,000) which is "specific" for schizophrenics but can also be found in stressed nonschizophrenic subjects (S-protein). This protein facilitates entry of tryptophan into cells. Recently these workers have reported that the tripeptide Thr-Val-Leu, a fragment of a larger endogenous protein, converts the S-protein to its nonschizophrenic form, and they now plan to administer this tripeptide to schizophrenic patients.

D. Cholecystokinin (CCK)

The role of CCK in the development of behavioral satiety serves as an example of the modulation of a specific homeostatic mechanism by a peptide hormone, and several excellent review articles have appeared on this subject (257,258). Porcine CCK is a 33-

membered amino acid chain. The C-terminal octapeptide of CCK (H-Asp- Tyr -Met-Gly-Trp-Met-Asp-Phe-NH$_2$) possess the full SO$_3$H biological activity of the hormone and is, in fact, about ten times more potent than the parent molecule on a molar basis (105). CCK causes gall bladder contraction and stimulates pancreatic secretion of glucagon and insulin (86). CCK is released when food enters the small intestine (186).

(1) Animal Studies

Gibbs and co-workers (93) first studied the effects of i.p. CCK on food consumption in the rat. The hormone produced a dose-dependent suppression of intake of both solid and liquid diets. Drinking behavior was unaffected (41,194); secretin had no anorectic effects. Further analysis (8,92) showed that CCK and the C-terminal octapeptide also elicited the complete behavioral sequence of satiety in rats with open gastric fistulas. These rats normally do not stop eating, presumably because of lack of gastric distention. CCK has also been shown to induce satiety in monkeys (94) and rabbits (121). Holt et al. (119) demonstrated that CCK does not produce bait shyness in rats, and therefore the effects on feeding behavior could not be explained by the possibility that CCK may have induced illness, but this finding has recently been questioned (57). Additional data strongly suggest the endogenous release of CCK as an important satiety signal under physiological conditions. Our group (201) have shown that small doses of the C-terminal octapeptide (1-100 µg/kg i.p.) significantly inhibits stress-induced eating in rats (Figure 2). This effect seems to be mediated via peripheral mechanisms, probably via vagally innervated structures (259). It is important to note, however, that CCK and fragments of CCK have been detected in human CSF (234).

(2) Human Studies

The studies cited above led two research groups to examine the effects of CCK on human food consumption. Sturdevant and Goetz (264) used a 20% pure CCK preparation in a double-blind study, and reported that after rapid i.v. injection, the hormone significantly reduced food intake whereas slow infusion of the hormone significantly increased food intake. Greenway and Bray (102) administered the C-terminal octapeptide of CCK (i.v. or s.c.) 10 or 20 minutes prior to a noontime liquid meal to 14 normal volunteers in a double-blind design. No significant differences in food intake were observed between CCK and vehicle-treated groups except for one

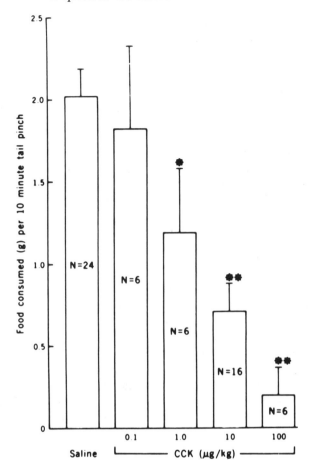

FIGURE 2   The effect of intraperitoneally administered CCK on tail pinch-induced eating in rats. Rats
were injected with 0.9 percent NaCl (pH 7.5), or CCK
(0.1 to 100 µg/kg). Five minutes later they were given
a 10-minute tail pinch (70 to 100 psi). Significance
was determined by Student's t-test, two-tailed; *P
< .05; **P < .001; N, number of animals. The thin
bars indicate standard error of mean. From Nemeroff, C.B., Osbahr, A.J., III, Bissette, G., Jahnke, G.,
Lipton, M.A., and Prange, A.J., Jr.: Cholecystokinin
inhibits tail pinch-induced eating in rats, *Science,* 200:
793-794, 1978, with permission. Copyright 1978 by
the American Association for the Advancement of
Science.

subject who consumed less after 20 ng/kg i.v.

These results cited above are disappointing but in view of potential therapeutic applications, further work on possible satiety effects of CCK in humans is needed. Larger doses of the peptide may be required. The highest dose utilized by Greenway and Bray (80 ng/kg) exerted no effect on stress-induced eating in rats (201) though a higher dose (100 μg/kg) almost totally abolished eating. Another important possibility to be examined is whether persons with anorexia—for example, anorexia nervosa patients—have high circulating levels of immunoreactive CCK. If CCK secretion is a physiological satiety signal, then disorders of CCK secretion may well play a role in some disorders of eating.

E. Neurotensin (NT)

NT is a tridecapeptide (pGlu-Leu-Tyr-Glu-Asn-Lys-Pro-Arg-Arg-Pro-Tyr-Ile-Leu-OH) (35-37). Unlike all other peptides mentioned in this review, it has not been administered to man. We have included it because much of our laboratory effort in recent years has been devoted to its study, because it appears to bear interesting relationships to two systems (dopaminergic and opioid) presumably involved in mental disorders, and because it appears to hold promise for investigation in mental disorders.

We have reviewed information pertaining to NT in detail 23, 203). In the present context we will include only material that has appeared more recently or is especially pertinent to the concept that NT may play a role in some mental disorders, notably schizophrenia.

(1) Isolation, Distribution and Binding

NT was originally detected during the isolation of substance P; a region of column effluent distinct from substance P when injected i.v. was found to produce hypotension, vasodilation, and cyanosis in rats (35,36). Characterization of the tridecapeptide was later accomplished by Carraway and Leeman (37).

A sensitive RIA for NT has been developed (39), and the distribution of the tridecapeptide has been studied. Two groups have described its distribution in rat brain (39,148). Immunoreactive NT concentrations are highest in the preoptic, septal, and hypothalamic areas, nucleus accumbens, amygdala, central gray of the midbrain, and nucleus interpeduncularis. Only 30% of immunoreactive NT in rat brain is present in the hypothalamus. Within the hypothalamus, the median eminence contains the highest concentration. Cerebrocortical regions and cerebellum contain very low concentrations. Radioimmunoassayable NT is found in high concentration in the small intestine and stomach (39).

Uhl and Snyder (279) have examined the regional and subcellular distribution of NT in calf brain. The heterogenous distribution of the peptide is similar to that observed in rat brain. Hypothalamic NT was found to be associated with the synaptosomal and microsomal fractions after density gradient centrifugation. Immunohistochemical methods have, for the most part, confirmed the NT distribution elucidated by RIA. The peptide has been visualized in the dog intestinal mucosa (206) and rat brain (278). In the rat CNS the tridecapeptide was localized by immunohistochemistry in a variety of structures including the substantia gelatinosa, central amygdaloid nucleus, median eminence, preoptic, and basal hypothalamic regions, and the adenohypophysis. Radioimmunoassay studies have now confirmed the presence of NT in gastrointestinal tissues (156).

Uhl et al. (277) have reported that ^{125}I-NT binds to rat and calf brain plasma membranes saturably, reversibly, and with high affinity. This binding is highest in thalamic, cerebrocortical, and hypothalamic brain regions. Similar results have been obtained with rat synaptosomal membrane preparations (144,155). These findings are consistent with the presence of physiologically meaningful NT receptors in the CNS. Recently Iversen et al. (128) have demonstrated NT release from slices of rat hypothalamus. This K^+-induced release was Ca^{++}dependent.

(2) General Effects

As mentioned above, the i.v. administration of NT causes hypotension, vasodilation, and cyanosis. These and other properties of NT have recently been surveyed (156,23).

(3) Endocrine Effects

NT administration *in vivo* causes hyperglycemia (32,36). Brown and Vale (32) confirmed the hyperglycemic effects of the peptide and also observed significant hypoinsulinemia and hyperglucagonemia after i.v. NT. Nagai and Frohman (196) have confirmed hyperglycemia and hyperglucagonemia after NT administration. Injections of NT into the lateral cerebral ventricles did not affect plasma glucose, insulin, or glucagon. They concluded that the pep-

Psychotropic Drug Research

tide probably acts on the pancreatic islets, the adrenal medulla, and the liver. In contrast to the findings of Leeman et al. (156), Rivier et al. (238) reported that i.v. NT induced a rise in plasma levels of PRL and GH. Carraway (35) reported that i.v. NT increases plasma levels of corticosterone, presumably by causing the release of ACTH from the adenohypophysis. Since morphine pretreatment blocks this effect, it is considered to be mediated via the CNS. This same group (178) reported that the tridecapeptide injected i.v. increases secretion of LH and FSH.

(4) Hypothermia after Central Administration

Since several studies have shown that peptides (e.g., TRH) can modify the sedative and hypothermic properties of barbiturates and other centrally acting depressants (21,31,228), we examined the effects of NT in this paradigm. The peripheral administration of NT (4.6 mg/kg i.p.) had no discernible effect on pentobarbital-induced narcosis and hypothermia. Intracisternally (i.c.) administered NT markedly enhanced the sedative and hypothermic effects observed after pentobarbital administration. In addition, centrally administered NT markedly enhanced the lethality of the barbiturate. The effects observed were dose-related (198).

Because of the apparent marked synergistic interaction with the barbiturate, the effect of i.c. NT (30 μg) on the disposition and metabolism of ^{3}H-pentobarbital was investigated (198). At this dose, which markedly potentiated the sedative effects of pentobarbital, NT significantly delayed the degradation and disposition of the barbiturate.

It is well recognized that hypothermia markedly alters drug metabolism (217). Since i.c. NT enhanced the depressant effects of pentobarbital and also decreased the rate of metabolism of the barbiturate, the effect of centrally administered NT on the decline in body temperature in a cold environment (4°C) was examined. This has been shown to be a sensitive measure of cold tolerance. NT administered i.c., markedly increased the rate and magnitude of the decline in colonic temperature (measured at 30 minute intervals) induced by two-hour cold exposure (22,198) in mice and rats. The hypothermic effect often showed an onset of action within one minute. This effect was clearly dose-related. The central administration of other endogenous peptides such as TRH, LHRH, MIF-I, SRIF, or Substance P had no effect in this paradigm.

In contrast to the effects obtained by i.c. administration, i.v.

administration of NT over a wide dose range (1 μg-10 mg/kg) was without effect on the rate of temperature loss in a cold environment (161,198).

The effects of NT (30 μg) on thermoregulatory processes of other mammalian and submammalian species have been studied. Centrally administered NT was found to be a potent hypothermic agent in the rat, hamster, gerbil, guinea pig, and monkey, but was without effect in the woodchuck, ground squirrel, rabbit, pigeon, frog, lizard, or fish (199, Figure 3).

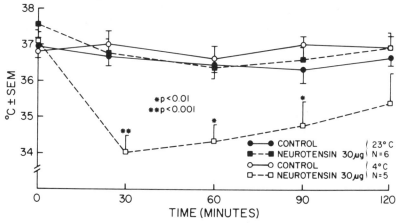

FIGURE 3 The effect of intracisternally administered neurotensin (30 μg) on the colonic temperature of adult male golden hamsters in an ambient temperature of 4°C or 23°C (Student's t-test, two-tailed).

In both series of experiments (pentobarbital test and the thermoregulatory paradigm), NT was inactive after peripheral administration. This suggests that the tridecapeptide penetrates the blood-brain barrier poorly if at all, that the CNS locus of action of this compound lies within the blood-brain barrier, and that the brain effects of this peptide are not mediated by peripheral processes.

Structure-activity studies have attempted to identify the "hypothermic" portion of the NT molecule (167). Substitution of single amino acids by their D-amino acid enantiomers in positions 6,7,8, and 11 does not significantly abolish the hypothermic properties of the peptide. However, the C-terminal pentapeptide is not hypothermic in the rat. Rivier et al. (239) reported that peptides structurally related to NT are hypothermic whereas those related to substance P are not. Bombesin (pGlu-Gln-Arg-Leu-Gly-Asn-Glu-Trp-Ala-Val-Gly-His-Leu-Met-NH$_2$), a tetradecapeptide isolated from frog skin, is 10,000 times more potent than NT in lowering the core temperature of rats exposed to *cold* (4°C); it is active in this paradigm in doses as low as 1 ng (i.c.) and is therefore one of the most potent peptides reported to exert CNS effects. We have confirmed these findings and have discovered several differences between NT and bombesin. When injected centrally into mice at *ambient* temperature (24°C) NT induces marked hypothermia; bombesin does not (64). Bombesin and NT apparently act differently to induce hypothermia. Thus naloxone or atropine pretreatment abolishes bombesin-induced hypothermia (M. Brown, personal communication) but does not affect NT-induced hypothermia.

(5) Analgesia after Central Administration

Of particular interest is the finding that NT possesses significant analgesic activity in mice (45). We have recently confirmed this finding and extended it to rats (204). On a molar basis, NT is a much more potent analgesic compound than met-enkephalin though it is clearly less potent than β-endorphin.

(6) Other Effects

The effect of a fixed dose of NT (30 μg i.c.v.) on the locomotor activity of adult rats has also been examined. Centrally administered NT induced significant reduction in locomotor activity when measured over a three hour period (198). NT also produces muscle relaxation after central administration in mice (208).

(7) Interactions with Acknowledged Transmitters

Other studies have been addressed to the interaction of NT with CNS neurotransmitter systems. Agents which block transmission of cholinergic, serotonergic, or noradrenergic systems do not antagonize the hypothermic properties of the tridecapeptide, but TRH, administered i.c., partially reverses this effect of NT (200). Treatments which reduce the functional activity of brain DA systems, such as DA depletion with 6-hydroxydopamine or haloperidol pretreatment, significantly potentiate NT-induced hypothermia.

Recently Malthe-Sorenssen et al. (179) have found that the intraventricular injection of NT increases the turnover of acetylcholine (ACh) in the diencephalon and decreased the ACh content of rat parietal cortex.

Peptides in Mental Disorders

(8) Neurotensin and Neuroleptics: A Comparison

Many of the NT effects listed above are reminiscent of the actions of acknowledged neuroleptic agents. Thus, neuroleptics are known to potentiate the effects of barbiturates (33), to produce hypothermia (33) and muscle relaxation (150), and to diminish spontaneous locomotor activity (132). In addition, effects of some of the neuroleptics, like some NT effects, are antagonized by TRH (31). A dissimilarity should be noted: neuroleptics, unlike NT, do not possess significant analgesic activity (46).

In light of the above findings we decided to compare the actions of NT and haloperidol, a potent antipsychotic and DA blocker, with only weak anticholinergic effects (164). The test system chosen was modification of the behavioral pattern produced in rats by the acute systemic administration of a potent DA releaser, d-amphetamine. Rats were prepared with indwelling cannulae placed bilaterally in each n. accumbens. One μl of NT, haloperidol, or vehicle solution was injected into each cannula immediately before d-amphetamine (2 mg/kg i.p.). Behavior of rats was subsequently observed in 10 second epochs for 30 seconds every 10 minutes for three hours, and scored by an observer ignorant of treatments using a standard behavioral checklist (81). NT (0.3 and 1 μg), like haloperidol (5 μg), significantly attenuated the forward locomotion elicited by amphetamine. NT (0.3 and 1 μg) also blocked amphetamine-induced rearing; haloperidol attenuated it but to no greater extent than its vehicle. Inhibition of locomotion and rearing by intra-accumbens injection of NT or haloperidol is consistent with the finding that it is in the n. accumbens where DA, released by amphetamine, elicits these behaviors (129,212).

Neither NT nor haloperidol inhibited the increased frequency of sniffing nor the insomnia produced by amphetamine. Thus, when injected into the nucleus accumbens, NT and haloperidol were similar in that they affected the same pair of amphetamine-induced behaviors while failing to affect two other amphetamine-induced behaviors. The two behaviors unaffected by these agents are thought to derive from the effects of amphetamines on sites other than or in addition to the n. accumbens (129,213). NT on both a weight and molar basis was more potent than haloperidol. The actions of NT cannot be regarded as nonspecific actions of peptides generally, for another endogenous peptide, SRIF, was ineffective.

Table VI summarizes the effects of centrally administered NT.

Psychotropic Drug Research

They not only show behavioral effects of this peptide but strongly indicate a negative effect on behaviors which are positively influenced by DA. Do these findings imply that NT may have properties like an endogenous neuroleptic? Alternatively does NT act in parallel as a system antagonistic to DA or as a facilitator of an antagonistic system? Although we have only begun exploration of NT mechanisms, preliminary experiments have shown that NT $(10^{-5} - 10^{-6}M)$ inhibits the binding of ^{3}H-spiroperidol to rat brain membranes rich in DA receptors (n. accumbens and n. caudatus). Whatever mechanisms may be involved, it appears clear from present data that NT exerts behavioral and physiological properties that resemble those of neuroleptics. We are currently examining the activity of NT in other standard screening tests for neuroleptics and are also attempting to assay NT levels in CSF and brain tissue from schizophrenic patients and sex-matched controls.

These findings concerning the pharmaco-behavioral profile of NT can be brought into clearer focus by considering the excellent discussion of Vereby et al. (25). These authors draw attention to the important relationships between opiate agonists (peptides and morphine) and brain DA systems. Many effects of opiate agonists are modified by pretreatment with DA agonists and antagonists. For example, both haloperidol and morphine antagonize the characteristic morphine withdrawal body shakes in rats and both also increases striatal DA turnover.

NT appears to be a compound that is at the interface of brain opiate and DA systems. Thus it possesses properties in common with both opiates (e.g. analgesia, hypothermia) and DA antagonists (e.g. amphetamine antagonism, potentiation of barbiturate sedation, diminished locomotor activity, etc.). This concatenation of findings tantalize the imagination concerning the possible role of NT in nervous and mental disorders.

VII. COMMENT

In animals at least some peptides exert behavioral effects that are not endocrine-dependent even when the peptides at issue are hormones. This has been established by either of two strategies: removing the target organs for the peptide under study and showing that the behavioral effect of the administered peptide is not lost; by administering the hormones secreted by these targets and showing that the behavioral effect does not occur. Whether these independent behavioral effects of peptides are physiological is more dif-

TABLE VI

A comparison of the pharmacological profile of acknowledged neuroleptics and centrally administered neurotensin.

Paradigm	NT	NT Dose Range	Maximum Effect	Neuro-leptics	Refs.
Potentiation of barbiturate sedation (mouse)	+	0.3-30 μg IC	↑ 275%	+	24 198 33
Hypothermia (mouse)	+	0.03-30 μg IC	-5°C	+	198 22 33
Muscle relaxation (mouse)	+	3.0-30 μg IC	Possible response, 52% of mice	+	208 33
Diminished Locomotor activity (rat)	+	30 μg ICV	↓ 50%	+	198 212
Blockade of amphetamine-induced locomotion and rearing (rat)	+	0.3-1 μg IC intra-accumbens	↓ 50% locomotion ↓100% rearing	+	164 213
Antagonism of hypothermia by TRH (10-80 μg IC) (rat)	+	30 μg IC	↓ 60%	+	164 213

TABLE VI (continued)

Antagonism of muscle relax-ation by TRH (30 µg IC) (mouse)	+	30 µg IC	Totally abolished	+	208 150
Analgesia - hot plate test (mouse)	+	2.5 µg IC	200% Reaction time	0	45

ficult to ascertain. Even when peptides are given directly into selected brain sites it is impossible to be sure that one has delivered physiological amounts to physiological sites of action. It is plausible, however, that at least some behavioral effects of some peptides are physiological. Phylogenetically some peptides, e.g., TRH, appear before their endocrine targets (104); some are widely distributed in brain (300); behavioral effects of a given peptide are often biologically harmonious with its endocrine effects (202).

The behavioral actions of peptides in man are more difficult to interpret than their behavioral actions in animals. It is especially difficult to establish that these effects are not reflections of endocrine effects. One cannot remove target organs. However, one can administer, say, the fast-acting thyroid hormone, L-triiodothyronine, and show that it fails to mimic the effects of TRH. If the time courses for producing a certain behavior of a peptide hormone and its evoked secretions are different, this is also a discriminating point. Additionally, one can mask the endocrine effects of some peptides. Thus, as indicated in our brief discussion of insulin, it is possible to prevent hypoglycemia by administering glucose. Finally, as noted in regard to ACTH, some congeners of natural peptides retain the behavioral effects of their parent compound but lack endocrine effects. Enough of these techniques have been applied to the study of enough peptides, we think, to conclude that in man, just as in animals, some endogenous peptides exert independent behavioral effects. The question of whether these effects are physiological or pharmacological is no farther advanced in human than in animal research.

Whatever the nature of the behavioral effects of peptides in man, what is their utility? At present the use of peptides is mainly heuristic rather than clinically practical. While TRH and MIF-I may have brief antidepressant effects, imipramine is a more reliable agent; while LHRH may enhance sexual receptivity, its effects in impotence are uncertain; while β-endorphin may raise pain threshold, morphine remains a preferred analgesic. Thus far the main value of peptide research in man is this: it has focused interest on a new class of compounds. Congeners of native peptides, rather than the authentic endogenous substances themselves, hold greatest therapeutic promise. Such compounds to be clinically useful would need several properties. Among such properties are resistance to rapid enzymatic degradation, freedom from unwanted endocrine effects, and increased penetration of the CNS after peripheral administration.

Psychotropic Drug Research

In man, certain peptides appear to elicit similar psychological responses. This suggests, of course, nonspecificity of action. A similar principle can be observed in animal behavioral studies. It is convenient to think, for example, that TRH antagonizes barbiturate sedation (31), that LHRH produces lordosis behavior (191, 192), and that ACTH delays extinction of conditioned avoidance. While these statements are true, it is also true that all three compounds (or their congeners), and others, delay extinction of conditioned avoidance (65). Furthermore, all these compounds, and others, antagonize barbiturate sedation (24). Lordosis behavior is produced relatively specifically by LHRH. However, TRH does affect this behavior; it antagonizes it. The principle of overlapping effects can be overstated. Potencies of peptides vary from one behavior to another and in some behavioral paradigms some peptides totally lack activity.

A problem that hampers the behavioral study of peptides in man, we think, is the lack of systematic measures for the dependent variables the peptides seem to affect. "Increased sense of well being, increased coping capacity" and kindred phrases appear repeatedly in anecdotal descriptions of responses of humans to peptide administration, but our assessment of changes in the parameters is presently crude. Standard rating scales have usually been employed. These have the single advantage of standardization; they have the liabilities of being oriented toward drug effects and specific diseases. Endogenous peptides are not drugs and they may well address normal adaptive functions more than the symptoms of diseases. One reason for entertaining this notion is the generalization that psychoactive drugs typically have only minor effects in normals while peptides may be quite active. The synthesis of appropriate congeners and the elaboration of appropriate measures would surely promote both the clinical application of peptides and our understanding of the full spectrum of their actions.

ACKNOWLEDGEMENTS

Preparation of this review was supported by NICHHD HD-03110, NIMH MH 32316, and NIMH MH 22536. We are grateful to Dorothy Yarbrough and Rosanne Altrows for help with this report.

REFERENCES

1. Akil, H., Richardson, D.E., Hughes, J., and Barchas, J.D.: Enkephalin-like material elevated in ventricular cerebrospinal fluid of pain pa-

tients after analgetic focal stimulation. *Science,* 201:436-465, 1978.

2. Akil, H., Watson, S.J., Berger, P.A., and Barchas, J.D.: Endorphins, β-LPH and ACTH: Biochemical, pharmacological and anatomical studies, In E. Costa and M. Trabucchi, (Eds.): *The Endorphins,* Raven Press, New York, 1978, pp. 125-139.

3. Akil, H., Watson, S.J., Sullivan, S., and Barchas, J.D.: Enkephalin-like material in normal human CSF: Measurements and levels. *Life Sci.* 23:121-126, 1978.

4. Altschule, M.D., Henneman, D.H., Holliday, P.D., and Goncz, R.M.: Carbohydrate metabolism in brain disease: VII. The effect of glutathione on carbohydrate intermediary metabolism in schizophrenic and manic-depressive psychoses. *A.M.A. Arch. Int. Med.* 99:22-27, 1957.

5. Altschule, M.D., Siegal, E.P., and Hennemann, D.H.: Blood glutathione level in mental disease before and after treatment. *Arch. Neurol. Psychiatry,* 67:64-68, 1952.

6. Anderson, M.S., Bowers, C.Y., Kastin, A.J., Schalch, D.S., Schally, A.V., Snyder, P.J., Utiger, R.D., Wilber, J.F., and Wise, A.J.: Synthetic thyrotropin-releasing hormone, a potent stimulator of thyrotropin secretion in man. *N. Eng. J. Med.,* 285:1279-1283, 1971.

7. Ant, M.: The nutritional factors in depressive states. *Am. J. Dig. Dis.,* 21:261-266, 1954.

8. Antin, J., Gibbs, J., Holt, J., Young, R.C., and Smith, G.P.: Cholecystokinin elicits the complete behavioral sequence of satiety in rats. *J. Comp. Physiol. Psychol.,* 89:784-790, 1975.

9. Appel, K.E., Farr, C.B., and Marshall, H.K.: Insulin in undernourished psychotic patients. *JAMA,* 90:1788, 1928; also *Arch. Neur. Psychiatry,* 21:149, 1929.

10. Assael, M., and Litiano, D.: Levels of glutathione in schizophrenic patients. *Dis. Nerv. Syst.,* 30:680-682, 1969.

11. Barak, A.J., Humoller, F.L., and Stevens, J.D.: Blood glutathione levels in the male schizophrenic patient. *Arch. Neurol. Psychiatry,* 80:237-240, 1958.

12. Barbeau, A.: Potentiation of levodopa effect by intravenous L-prolyl-L-leucyl-glycine amide in men. *Lancet,* ii:683-689, 1975.

13. Becker: Insulin bei nahrungverwiegernden Geisteskranken. *Psychiatry-Neurol. Woch.,* 30:547, 1928.

14. Benkert, O.: Studies on pituitary hormones and releasing hormones in depression and sexual impotence, In W.H. Gispen, Tj.B. van Wimersma Greidanus, B. Bohus and D. de Wied, (Eds.): *Hormones, Homeostasis and the Brain. Progress in Brain Research,* 42, Elsevier, Amsterdam, 1975, pp. 25-36.

15. Benkert, O., Gordon, A., and Martschke, D.: The comparison of thyrotropin releasing hormone, luteinizing hormone-releasing hormone and placebo in depressive patients using a double-blind cross-over technique. *Psychopharmacologia (Berl.)* 40:191-198, 1974.

Psychotropic Drug Research

16. Bennett, A.E., and Semrad, E.V.: Value of insulin treatment in undernourished psychiatric patients. *Am. J. Psychol.,* 92:1425-1431, 1936.
17. Betts, T.A., Smith, J., Pidd, S., Mackintosh, J., Harvey, P., and Funicane, J.: The effects of thyrotropin-releasing hormone on measures of mood in normal women. *Br. J. Clin. Pharmacol.,* 3:469-473, 1976.
18. Beutler, E.: Disorders in glutathione metabolism. *Life Sci.,* 16:1499-1506, 1977.
19. Bigelow, L.G., Gillin, J.C., Semal, C., and Wyatt, R.J.: Thyrotropin releasing hormone in chronic schizophrenia. *Lancet,* ii:869-870, 1975.
20. Bird, E.D., Chieppa, S.A., and Fink, G.: Brain immunoreactive gonadotropin-releasing hormone in Huntington's chorea and in nonchoreic subjects. *Nature,* 260:536-538, 1976.
21. Bissette, G., Nemeroff, C.B., Loosen, P.J., Prange, A.J., Jr., and Lipton, M.A.: Comparison of the analeptic potency of TRH, LHRH, ACTH and related peptides. *Pharmacol. Biochem. Behav.,* 5 (Suppl. 1):135-138.
22. Bissette, G., Nemeroff, C.B., Loosen, P.T., Prange, A.J., Jr., and Lipton, M.A.: Hypothermia and intolerance to cold induced by intracisternal administration of the hypothalamic peptide neurotensin. *Nature,* 262:607-609, 1976.
23. Bissette, G., Manberg, P.J., Nemeroff, C.B. and Prange, A.J., Jr.: Neurotensin, a biologically active peptide. *Life Sci.,* 23:2173-2182, 1978.
24. Bissette, G., Nemeroff, C.B., Loosen, P.T., Breese, G.R., Lipton, M.A., and Prange, A.J., Jr.: Modification of pentobarbital-induced sedation by natural and synthetic peptides. *Neuropharmacology,* 17: 229-237, 1978.
25. Bloom, F.E., Rossier, J., Battenburg, E.L.F., Bayon, A., French, E., Henriksen, S.J., Siggins, G.R., Segal, D., Browne, R., Ling, N., and Guillemin, R.: β-endorphin: Cellular localization, electrophysiological and behavioral effects. In E. Costa and M. Trabucchi (Eds.): *The Endorphins,* Raven Press, New York, 1978, pp. 89-109.
26. Blume, A.J., Sharr, J., Finberg, J.P.M., and Spector, S.S.: Binding of the endogenous nonpeptide morphine-like compound to opiate receptors. *Proc. Natl. Acad. Sci.,* 74 (11):4927-4931, 1977.
27. Bohus, B.: Pituitary peptides and adaptive autonomic responses. In W.H. Gispen, T.B., van Wimersma Greidanus, B. Bohus. (Eds.): *Hormones, Homeostasis and the Brain,* Elsevier, Amsterdam, 1975.
28. Bowers, C.Y., Friesen, N.G., Hwang, P., Guyda, H.Y. and Folkers, K.: Prolactin and thyrotropin release in man by synthetic pyroglutamyl-histidyl-prolinamide. *Biochem. Biophys. Res. Commun.,* 45:1033-1041, 1971.
29. Brambilla, F., Rovere, C., Guastalla, A., Guerrini, A., and Riggi, F.: Gonadotropin response to synthetic gonadotropin hormone-releasing

hormone (GRH) in chronic schizophrenia. *Acta Psychiatry Scand.,* 54:131-145, 1976.

30. Brazeau, P., Vale, W., Burgus, R., Ling, N., Butcher, M., Rivier, J., and Guillemin, R.: Hypothalamic polypeptide that inhibits the secretion of immunoreactive pituitary growth hormone. *Science,* 179:77-79, 1973.
31. Breese, G.R., Cott, J.M., Cooper, B.R., Prange, A.J., Jr., Lipton, M.A., and Plotnikoff, N.P.: Effects of thyrotropin-releasing hormone (TRH) on the actions of pentobarbital and other centrally acting drugs. *J. Pharmacol. Exp. Ther.,* 193:11-22, 1975.
32. Brown, M., and Vale, W.: Effects of neurotensin and substance P on plasma insulin, glucagon, and glucose levels. *Endocrinology,* 98:819-821, 1976.
33. Byck, R.: Drugs and the treatment of psychiatric disorders, In L. Goodman and A. Gilman (Eds.): *The Pharmacological Basis of Therapeutics,* MacMillan, New York, 1975, pp. 152-200.
34. Campbell, M., Hollander, C.S., Ferris, S., and Greene, L.W.: Response to TRH stimulation in young psychotic children: A pilot study. *Psychoneuroendocrinology,* 2:195-202, 1978.
35. Carraway, R.E.: The isolation, chemical and pharmacological characterization, and the synthesis of a new hypothesive peptide: neurotensin, Ph.D. dissertation, Brandeis University, 1972.
36. Carraway, R.E., and Leeman, S.E.: The isolation of a new hypotensive peptide, neurotensin, from bovine hypothalamus. *J. Biol. Chem.,* 248:6854-6861, 1973.
37. Carraway, R.E., and Leeman, S.E.: The amino acid sequence of a hypothalamic peptide, neurotensin. *J. Biol. Chem.,* 250:1907-1918, 1975.
38. Carraway, R.E., Demers, L.M., and Leeman, S.E.: Hyperglycemic effect of neurotensin, a hypothalamic peptide. *Endocrinology,* 99:1452-1462, 1976.
39. Carraway, R.E., and Leeman, S.E.: Characterization of radioimmunoassayable neurotensin in the rat. *J. Biol. Chem.,* 254:7045-7052, 1976.
40. Carroll, B.J., and Mendels, J.: Neuroendocrine regulation in affective disorders, In E. J. Sachar (Ed.): *Hormones, Behavior, and Psychopathology,* Raven Press, New York, 1976, pp. 41-68.
41. Catlin, D.H., Hui, K.K., Loh, H.H., and Li, C.N.: Pharmacologic activity of β-endorphin in men. *Comm. Psychopharmacol.,* 1:493-500, 1977.
42. Chase, T.N., Woods, A.C., Lipton, M.A., and Morris, C.E.: Hypothalamic releasing factors and Parkinson's disease. *Arch. Neurol.,* 31:55-56, 1974.
43. Chazot, G., Chalumeau, A., Aimard, G., Mornex, R., Garde, A., Schott, B., and Girard, P.F.: Thyrotropin releasing hormone and depressive states: From agroagonines to TRH. *Lyon Med.* 231:831-836, 1974.

Psychotropic Drug Research

44. Clark, M.S., Parades, A., Costiloe, J.P., and Wood, F.: Synthetic thyroid releasing hormone (TRH) administered orally to chronic schizophrenic patients. *Psychopharmacol. Commun.*, 1(2):191-200, 1975.

45. Clineschmidt, B.V., and McGuffin, J.C.: Neurotensin administered intracisternally inhibits responsiveness of mice to noxious stimuli. *Europ. J. Pharmacol.*, 46:395-396, 1977.

46. Cocchi, D., Santagostrono, A., Gil-Ad, I., Ferri, S., and Muller, E.E.: Leu-enkephalin-stimulated growth hormone and prolactin release in the rat: Comparison with the effect of morphine. *Life Sci.*, 20:2041-2046, 1977.

47. Coppen, A., Montgomery, S., Peet, M., and Bailey, J.: Thyrotropin-releasing hormone in the treatment of depression. *Lancet*, ii:433-434, 1974.

48. Costa, E., and Trabucchi, M. (Eds.) : *The Endorphins*, Raven Press, New York, 1978.

49. Cotzias, G.C., Von Woert, M.H., and Schiffer, L.M.: Aromatic amino acids and modification of Parkinsonism. *N. Eng. J. Med.*, 276:374-379, 1967.

50. Cotzias, G.C., Paparasiliou, P.S., and Rosal, V.L.F.: Apomorphines, somatostatin and Parkinson's disease. In P. Deniker, C. Radouco-Thomas, and A. Killeneuve (Eds.): *Neuropsychopharmacology*, Pergamon Press, Oxford, New York, 1978, pp. 703-708.

51. Daughaday, W.H.: The adenohypophysis. In R. H. Williams (Ed.) : *Textbook of Endocrinology*, W.B. Saunders Co., Philadelphia, 1974.

52. Davis, G.C., Bunney, W.E., Jr., Defraites, E.G., Kleinman, J.E., van Kammen, D.P., and Wyatt, R.J.: Intravenous naloxone administration in schizophrenia and affective illness. *Science*, 197:74-77, 1977.

53. Davis, G.C., Duncan, W.C., Gillin, J.C., and Bunney, W.E., Jr.: Failure of naloxone to affect human sleep. *Comm. Psychopharmacol.*, 1:489-492, 1977.

54. Davis, K.L., Hollister, L.E., and Berger, P.A.: Thyrotropin-releasing hormones in schizophrenia. *Am. J. Psychiatry*, 132(9):951-953, 1975.

55. Delitala, G., Masala, A., Alagna, S., and Litti, G.: Luteinizing hormone, folicle stimulating hormone and testosterone in normal and impotent men following LH-RH and HLG stimulation. *Clin. Endocr.*, 6:11-15, 1977.

56. Deniker, P., Ginestet, D., Loo, H., Zaririan, E., and Cottereau, M.J.: Preliminary study of the action of hypothalamic thyrostimulin (TRH) in depressive states. *Ann. Med. Psychol.*, 1(2):249-255, 1974.

57. Deutsch, J.A., and Hardy, W.T.: Cholecystokinin produces bait shyness in rats. *Nature*, 266:196, 1976.

58. de Wied, D.: Effects of peptide hormones on behavior. In W.F. Ganong, and L. Martini (Eds.) : *Frontiers in Neuroendocrinology 1969*, Oxford University Press, London, 1969, pp. 97-140.

59. de Wied, D.: Long-term effect of vasopressin on the maintenance of a conditioned avoidance response in rats. *Nature*, 232:58-60, 1971.

60. de Wied, D.: Pituitary-adrenal hormones and behavior. In G.B.A. Stoelings, ten van den Werff, J.J. Bosch (Eds.) : *Normal and Abnormal Development of Brain and Behavior,* Laden University Press, Laden, The Netherlands, 1971.
61. de Wied, D.: The role of the posterior pituitary and its peptides on the maintenance of conditioned avoidance behavior. In K. Lissak, (Ed.) : *Hormones and Brain Function,* Plenum Press, New York, 1973.
62. de Wied, D.: Pituitary-adrenal system hormones and behavior. In F.O. Schmitt and F.G. Worden (Eds.) : *The Neurosciences Third Study Program,* MIT Press, Cambridge, 1974.
63. de Wied, D., Bohus, B., and van Wimersa Greidanus, T.B.: The hypothalamoneurophypophyseal system and the preservation of conditioned avoidance behavior in rats. In D.E. Swaab and J.P. Schade (Eds.) : *Integrative Hypothalamic Activity, Progress in Brain Research,* Vol. 42, Elsevier, Amsterdam, 1974, pp. 417-427.
64. de Wied, D., Bohus, B., and Urban, I.: Pituitary peptides and memory. In R. Walter and J. Meicnhofer (Eds.) : *Peptides: Chemistry Structure and Biology,* Ann Arbor Publishers, Ann Arbor, Mich., 1975.
65. de Wied, D., Witter, A., and Greven, H.M.: Behaviorally active ACTH analogues. *Biochem. Pharmacol.,* 24:1463-1468, 1975.
66. de Wied, D., and Gispen, W.H.: Behavioral effects of peptides. In H. Gainer (Ed.): *Peptides in Neurobiology,* Plenum Press, New York, 1977.
67. de Wied, D., Bohus, B., van Ree, J.M., Kovacs, G.L., and Greven, H.M.: Neuroleptic-like activity of Des-Tyr[1]-γ-endorphin in rats. *Lancet,* i:1046, 1978.
68. de Wied, D., and van Ree, J.M.: Endorphine and schizophrenia. *Proc. 2nd World Congress of Biological Psychiatry,* 1978, p. 100.
69. Dimitrikoudi, M., Hanson-Norty, E., and Jenner, F.A.: TRH in psychoses. *Lancet,* i:456, 1974.
70. Drayson, A.M.: TRH in cyclical psychoses. *Lancet,* ii:312, 1974.
71. Easterday, O.D., Featherstone, R.M., Gottlieb, J.S., Nusser, M.L., and Hogg, R.V.: Blood glutathione, lactic acid, and pyruvic acid relationships in schizophrenia. *Arch. Neurol. Psychiatry,* 68:48-57, 1953.
72. Eddy, N.B., and May, E.L.: Origin and history of antagonists. In M.C. Branola, L.S. Hanes, E.L. May, J.P. Smith and E.D. Villaneal (Eds.): *Narcotic Antagonists,* Adv. Biochem. Psychopharmacol., 8, Raven Press, New York, 1974, pp. 9-11.
73. Efendic, S., and Luft, R.: Studies on the mechanism of somatostatin action on insulin release in man. *Acta Endocr.,* 78:516-523, 1975.
74. Ehrensing, R.H., and Kastin, A.J.: Melanocyte-stimulating hormone-release inhibiting hormone as an antidepressant. *Arch. Gen. Psychiatry,* 30:63-65, 1974.
75. Ehrensing, R.H., Kastin, A.J., Schalch, D.S., Friesen, H.G., Vargas, J.R., and Schally, A.V.: Affective state and thyrotropin and prolactin

173

responses after repeated injections of thyrotropin-releasing hormone in depressed patients. *Am. J. Psychiatry,* 131(6):714-718, 1974.

76. Ehrensing, R.H., and Kastin, A.J.: Dose-related biphasic effect of prolyl-leucyl-glycinamide (MIF-I) in depression. *Am. J. Psychiatry,* 135:562-566, 1978.

77. Elde, R., and Hokfelt, T.: Distribution of hypothalamic hormones and other peptides in the brain. In W.F. Ganong and L. Martini (Eds.): *Frontiers in Neuroendocrinology,* Vol. 5, Raven Press, New York, 1978, pp. 1-33.

78. Ellman, G.L., and Gan, G.L.: Erythrocyte glutathione levels in patients of a mental hospital. *Nature,* 202:904, 1964.

79. Endroczi, E., Lissak, K., Fekete, T., and de Wied, D.: Effects of ACTH on EEG habituation in human subjects. In D. de Wied, and J.A.W.M. Weijnen (Eds.): *Progress in Brain Research,* Vol. 32, Elsevier, Amsterdam, 1970, pp. 254-262.

80. Endroczi, E.: Pavlovian conditioning and adaptive hormones. In S. Levine (Ed.): *Hormones and Behavior,* Academic Press, New York, 1972, pp. 173-208.

81. Ervin, G.N., Fink, J.S., Young, R.C., and Smith, G. P.: Differential behavioral responses to L-dopa after anterolateral or posterolateral hypothalamic injections of 6-hydroxydopamine. *Brain Res.,* 132:507-520, 1977.

82. Ettigi, P.G., and Brown, G.: TSH and LH responses in subtypes of depression. *Annual Meeting, Am. Psychosomatic Society,* Washington, D.C., March 1978.

83. Evans, L.E.J., Hunter, P., Hall, R., Johnston, M., and Roy, V.M.: A double-blind trial of intravenous thyrotropin-releasing hormone in the treatment of reactive depression. *Br. J. Psychiatry,* 127:227-230, 1975.

84. Fleischer, N., Burgus, R., Vale, W., Dunn, T., and Guillemin, R.: Preliminary observations on the effect of synthetic thyrotropin releasing factor on plasma thyrotropin levels in man. *J. Clin. Endocr. Metab.,* 31:109-112, 1970.

85. Forizs, L., Vitols, E., and Vitols, M.: Combined pitressin and electric shock in schizophrenia. *Dis. Nerv. Syst.,* 15:176-179, 1954.

86. Frame, C.M., Davidson, M.B., and Sturdevant, R.A.L.: Effects of the octapeptide of cholecystokinin on insulin and glucagon secretion in the dog. *Endocrinology.* 97:549-553, 1975.

87. Frederickson, R.C., Burgus, V., Harrell, C.E., and Edwards, J.D.: Dual actions of substance P on nocioception: Possible role of endogenous opioids. *Science,* 199:1359-1362, 1978.

88. Furlong, F.W., Brown, G.M., and Beeching, M.F.: Thyrotropin-releasing hormone: Differential antidepressant and endocrinological effects. *Am. J. Psychiatry.* 133:1187-1190, 1976.

89. Gaillard, A.W.K., and Sanders, A.F.: Some effects of $ACTH_{4-10}$ on performance during a serial reaction task. *Psychopharmacologia,* 42:

201-208, 1975.

90. Gerich, J.E., Lorenzi, M., Bier, D.M., Schneider, V., Tsalikian, E., Karam, J.H., and Forsham, P.H.: Prevention of human diabetic ketoacidosis by somatostatin. *New Eng. J. Med.,* 292(19):985-989, 1975.

91. Gerstenbrand, F., Binder, H., Kozma, C., Pusch, S., and Reisner, T.: Infusionstherapie mit MIF (melanocyte inhibiting factor) beim Parkinson-syndrome. *Wiener Klin. Wschr.,* 24:822-823, 1975.

92. Gibbs, J., Young, R.C., and Smith, G.P.: Cholecystokinin decreases food intake in rats. *J. Comp. Physiol. Psychol.,* 84:488-495, 1973.

93. Gibbs, J., Young, R.C., and Smith, G.P.: Cholecystokinin elicits satiety in rats with open gastric fistulas. *Nature (London),* 245:323-325, 1973.

94. Gibbs, J., Falasco, J.D., and McHugh, P.R.: Cholecystokinin-decreased food intake in rhesus monkeys. *Am. J. Physiol.,* 230:15-18, 1976.

95. Gold, P.W., Goodwin, F.K., Wehr, T., and Rebar, R.: Pituitary thyrotropin response to thyrotropin-releasing hormone in affective illness: Relationship to spinal fluid amine metabolites. *Am. J. Psychiatry,* 134(9):1028-1031, 1977.

96. Gold, P.W., Goodwin, F.K., and Reus, V.I.: Vasopressin in affective illness. *Lancet,* i:1233-1236, 1978.

97. Goldstein, A., and Hilgard, E.R.: Failure of the opiate antagonist naloxone to modify hypnotic analgesia. *Proc. Natl. Acad. Sci.,* 72: 2041-2043, 1975.

98. Goldstein, A.: Opioid peptides in pituitary and brain. *Science,* 193: 1081-1086, 1976.

99. Goldstein, A., and Hansteen, R.W.: Evidence against involvement of endorphins in sexual arousal and orgasm in men. *Arch. Gen. Psychiatry,* 34:1179-1180, 1977.

100. Gottlieb, J.S., and Frohman, C.E.: A neuropolypeptide, based on biochemical phenomenology, possibly effective in treatment of schizophrenia. In W.E. Fann, I. Karacan, A.D. Pokorny and R.L. Williams (Eds.): *Phenomenology and Treatment of Schizophrenia,* Spectrum Publ. Inc., New York, 1978, pp. 455-465.

101. Goujet, M.A., Simon, P., Chermat, R., and Boissier, J.R.: Profil de la TRH en psychopharmacologie experimentale. *Psychopharmacologia (Berl),* 45:87-92, 1975.

102. Greenway, F.L., and Bray, G.A.: Cholecystokinin and satiety. *Life Sci.,* 21:769-772, 1978.

103. Gregoire, F., Brauman, H., de Buck, R., and Corvilain, J.: Hormone release in depressed patients before and after recovery. *Psychoneuroendocrinology,* 2:303-312, 1977.

104. Grimm-Jørgensen, Y., and McKelvy, J.F.: Immunoreactive thyrotropin releasing factor in gastropod circumoesophageal ganglia. *Nature (London),* 254:620, 1975.

Psychotropic Drug Research

105. Grossman, M.I.: Gastrointestinal hormones. *Viewpoints Digest Dis.,* 2:1-4, 1970.
106. Guillemin, R.: Peptides in the brain: The new endocrinology of the neuron. *Science,* 202:390-402, 1978.
107. Gunne, L.M., Lindstrom, L., and Terenius, L.: Naloxone-induced reversal of schizophrenic hallucinations. *J. Neur. Trans.* 40:13-19, 1977.
108. Haack, H.: Insulin bei nahrungsverweigernden Geisteskranken. *Psychiat. Neurol. Woch.,* 31:195, 1929.
109. Haigler, E.D., Jr., Pittman, J.A., Jr., Hershman, J.M., and Baugh, C.M.: Direct evaluation of pituitary thyrotropin reserve utilizing synthetic thyrotropin releasing hormone. *J. Clin. Endocr. Metab.,* 33:573, 1971.
110. Hall, R., Hunter, P.R., Price, J.S., and Mountjoy, C.Q. Thyrotropin-releasing hormone in depression. *Lancet,* i:162, 1975.
111. Halmi, K.A.: Selective pituitary deficiency in anorexia nervosa. In E. J. Sachar (Ed.): *Hormones, Behavior and Psychopathology,* Raven Press, New York, 1976, pp. 285-290.
112. Hamilton, M.: A rating scale for depression. *J. Neurol. Neurosurg. Psychiatry,* 23:56-62, 1960.
113. Havrankova, J., Roth, J., and Brownstein, M.: Insulin receptors are widely distributed in the CNS of the rat. *Nature,* 272:827-829, 1978.
114. Henderson, W.G., Tourtellotte, W.W., Potnin, A.R., and Rose, A.S.: Methodology for analyzing clinical neurological data: ACTH in multiple sclerosis. *Clin. Pharm. Therap.,* 24:146-153, 1978.
115. Henneman, D.H., and Goncz, R.M.: Carbohydrate metabolism in brain disease: II. Glucose metabolism in schizophrenic, manic-depressive, and involutional psychoses. *AMA Arch. Int. Med.,* 94:402-416, 1954.
116. Herz, A., Blasig, J., Emrich, H.M., Cording, G., Piree, S., Kolling, A., and von Zeussen, D.: Is there some indication from behavioral effects of endorphins for their involvement in psychiatric disorders? In E. Costa and M. Trabucchi, (Eds.): *The Endorphins,* Raven Press, New York, 1978, pp. 333-339.
117. Hokfelt, T., Efendic, S., Hellerstrom, C., Johanssen, O., Witt, R., and Arimura, A.: Cellular localization of somatostatin in endocrine-like cells and neurons of the rat with special references to the A_1-cells of the pancreatic islets and to the hypothalamus. *Acta Endocr.,* 80 (Suppl 200):1-41, 1975.
118. Hollister, L.E., Berger, P., Ogle, F.L., Arnold, R.C., and Johnson, A.: Protirelin (TRH) in depression. *Arch. Gen. Psychiatry,* 31:468-470, 1974.
119. Holt, J., Antin, J., Gibbs, J.,and Young, R.C.: Cholecystokinin does not produce bait shyness in rats. *Physiol. Behav.,* 12:497-498, 1974.
120. Hisobuchi, Y., and Li, C.H.: The analgesic activity of human β-endorphin in man. *Comm. Psychopharmacol.,* 2:33-37, 1978.
121. Houpt, T.R., Anika, S.M., and Wolff, N.C.: Satiety effects of chol-

Peptides in Mental Disorders

ecystokinin and caerolin in rabbits. *Am. J. Physiol.,* 235:1223-1228, 1974.

122. Huey, L.Y., Janowsky, D.S., Mandell, A.J., Judd, L.L., and Pendery, M.: Preliminary studies on the use of thyrotropin releasing hormone in manic states, depression, and the dysphoria of alcohol withdrawal. *Psychopharmacol. Bull.,* 11(1):24-27, 1975.

123. Huidobro-Toro, J.P., Scotti de Carolis, A., and Longo, V.G.: Action of two hypothalamic factors (TRH, MIF) and of angiotensin II on the behavioral effects of L-dopa and 5-hydroxytryptophan in mice. *Pharmacol. Biochem. Behav.,* 2:105-109, 1974.

124. Hutton, W.N.: Thyrotropin-releasing hormone in depression. *Lancet,* ii:53, 1974.

125. Inanaga, K., Nakano, T., and Nagato, T.: Effects of thyrotropin releasing hormone in schizophrenia. *Kurume Med. J.,* 22:159-168, 1975.

126. Inanaga, K., Nakano, T., Nagato, T., Tanaka, M., and Ogawa, N.: Behavioral effects of protirelin in schizophrenia. *Arch. Gen. Psychiatry,* 35:1011-1014, 1978.

127. Itil, T.M., Patterson, C.D., Polvan, N., Bigelow, A., and Bergey, B.: Clinical and CNS effects of oral and I.V. thyrotropin-releasing hormone in depressed patients. *Dis. Nerv. Syst.,* 36(9):529-536, 1975.

128. Iversen, L.L., Iversen, S.D., Bloom, F.E., Douglas, C., Brown, M., and Vale, W.: Calcium-dependent release of somatostatin and neurotensin from rat brain in vitro. *Nature,* 273:161-163, 1978.

129. Jackson, D.M., Anden, N.E., and Dahlstrom, A.A.: A functional effect of dopamine in the nucleus accumbens and in some other dopamine rich parts of the rat brain. *Psychopharmacologia (Berl.),* 41:175, 1975.

130. Jacob, E., and Doussinet, P.: Traitement insulinique d'un groupe de cetoses en pathologie mentale. *Bull. Gen. Therap.,* 184:12, 1933.

131. Jenniewic, N., Brown, G.M., Garfinkel, P.E., and Moldofsky, H.: Hypothalamic function as related to body weight and body fat in anorexia nervosa. *Psychoso. Med.,* XL:187-198, 1978.

132. Jalfrie, M., and Haefely, W.: Effects of centrally acting agents in rats after intraventricular injections of 6-hydroxydopamine. In S.E. Malmfors and H. Thoehen (Eds.), *6-Hydroxydopamine and Catecholamine Neurons,* American Elsevier, New York, 1971.

133. Janowsky, D.S., Segal, D., Bloom, F., Abrams, A., and Guillemin, R.: Lack of effect of naloxone on schizophrenic symptoms. *Am. J. Psychiatry.* 134:926-927, 1977.

134. Kastin, A.J., Miller, L.H. Gonzales-Barcena, D., Hawley, W.D., Dyster-Aas, K., Schally, A.V., Velasco de Parra, M.L., and Velasco, M.: Psychophysiologic correlates of MSH in man. *Physiol. Behav.,* 7: 893-896, 1971.

135. Kastin, A.J., and Barbeau, A.: Preliminary clinical studies with L-prolyl-L-leucyl-glycine amide in Parkinson's disease. *CMA J.,* 107:

177

1079-1081, 1972.

136. Kastin, A.J., Ehrensing, R.H., Schalch, D.S., and Anderson, M.S.: Improvement in mental depression with decreased thyrotropin response after administration of thyrotropin-releasing hormone. *Lancet,* ii:740-742, 1972.

137. Kastin, A.M., Plotnikoff, N.P., and Sandman, C.A.: The effects of MSH and MIF on the brain. In W.E. Stumpf, and L.D. Grant (Eds.): *Anatomical Neuroendocrinology,* S. Karger, Basel, 1975.

138. Kastin, A.J., Sandman, C.A., Stratton, L.O., Schally, A.V., and Miller, L.H.: Behavioral and electrographic changes in rat and man after MSH. In W.H. Gispen, Tj.B. van Wimersma Greidanus, B. Bohus and D. de Wied (Eds.): *Hormones, Homeostasis and the Brain, Progress in Brain Research,* Elsevier, Amsterdam, 1975, Vol. 42, pp. 143-150.

139. Kastin, A.J., Plotnikoff, N.P., Schally, A.V., and Sandman, C.A.: Endocrine and CNS effects of hypothalamic peptides and MSH. In S. Ehrenpreis and I.J. Kopin (Eds.): *Reviews of Neuroscience 2,* Raven Press, New York, 1976.

140. Katz, J.L., Boyar, R.M., Weiner, H., Gorzynski, G., Roffwarg, H., and Hellman, L.: Toward an elucidation of the psychoendocrinology of anorexia nervosa. In E.J. Sachar (Ed.): *Hormones, Behavior and Psychopathology.* Raven Press, New York, 1976, pp. 263-284.

141. Kieley, W.F., Adrian, A.D., Lee, J.H., and Nicoloff, J.T.: Therapeutic failure of oral TRH in depression. *Psychoso. Med.,* 38:233-241, 1976.

142. Kirkegaard, C., Norlem, N., Lauridsen, U.B., Bjorum, N., and Christiansen, C.: Protirelin stimulation test and thyroid function during treatment of depression. *Arch. Gen. Psychiatry.* 32:1115-1118, 1975.

143. Kirkegaard, C. Bjorum, N., Cohn, D., and Lauridsen, U.B.: TRH stimulation test in manic depressive disease. *Arch. Gen. Psychiatry.* 35:1017-1023, 1978.

144. Kitabgi, P., Carraway, R., van Rietschoten, J., Graver, C., Morgat, J.C., Menez, A., Leeman, S., and Freychet, P.: Neurotensin: Specific binding to synaptic membranes from rat brain. *Proc. Nat. Acad. Sci.,* 74:1846-1850, 1977.

145. Kleeman, C.R., and Vorhen, H.: Water metabolism and the neurophypophyseal hormones. In P.K. Bondy and L.E. Rosenberg (Eds.): *Duncan's Diseases of Metabolism: Endocrinology,* 7th Edition, W.B. Saunders, Co., Philadelphia, 1974.

146. Klein, R.: The effects of ACTH and corticosteroids in epileptiform disorders. In D. de Wied and J.A.W.M. Weijnen (Eds.): *Pituitary, Adrenal and The Brain, Progress in Brain Research,* Vol. 32, Elsevier, Amsterdam, 1970, pp. 263-269.

147. Kline, N.S., Li, C.H., Lehmann, H.E., Lajtha, A., Laski, E., and Cooper, T.: β-endorphin-induced changes in schizophrenic and depressed patients. *Arch. Gen. Psychiatry.* 34:1111-1113, 1977.

148. Kobayashi, R.N., Brown, M., and Vale, W.: Regional distribution of

neurotensin and somatostatin in rat brain. *Brain Res.,* 126:584-588, 1977.

149. Krieger, P.T., Liotta, A., and Brownstein, M.J.: Presence of corticotropin in brain of normal and hypophysectomized rats. *Proc. Natl. Acad. Sci.,* 74:648-652, 1977.

150. Kruse, H.: Thyrotropin-releasing hormone: Interaction with clorpromazine in mice, rats and rabbits. *J. Pharmacol. (Paris),* 6:249-268,1975.

151. Kurland, A.A., McCabe, O.L., Hanlon, T.E., and Sullivan, D.: The treatment of preceptual disturbances in schizophrenia with naloxone hydrochloride. *Am. J. Psychiatry,* 134:12, 1977.

152. La Ferla, T.T., Anderson, D.L., and Schalch, D.S.: Psychoendocrine response to sexual arousal in human males. *Psychoso. Med.,* 40:166-172, 1978.

153. Lakke, J.P.W.F., van Praag, H.M., van Twisk, R., Doorenbos, H., and Witt, F.G.J.: Effects of administration of thyrotropin releasing hormone in Parkinsonism. *Clin. Neurol. Neurosurg.,* 3/4:1-5, 1974.

154. Lamberg, B.A., Linnoila, M., Fogelholm, R., Olkinuora, M., Kohlainer, P., and Saarinen, P.: The effect of psychotropin drugs on the TSH-response to thyroliberin (TRH). *Neuroendocrinology,* 24:96-97, 1977.

155. Lazarus, L.H., Brown, M., and Perrin, M.H.: Distribution, localization and characteristics of neurotensin binding sites in the rat brain, *Neuropharmacology,* 16:625-629, 1977.

156. Leeman, S.E., Mroz, E.A. and Carraway, R.E.: Substance P and neurotensin. In H.E. Gainor (Ed.): *Peptides in Neurobiology,* Plenum Press, New York, 1977, pp. 99-144.

157. Leppaluoto, T., Rapeli, M., Varis, R. and Ranta, T.: Secretion of anterior pituitary hormones in man: Effects of ethyl alcohol. *Acta Physiol. Scand.,* 95:400-406, 1975.

158. Levine, J.D., Gordon, N.C., Jones, R.T., and Fieldo, H.C.: The narcotic antagonist naloxone enhances clinical pain. *Nature,* 272:826-827, 1978.

159. Lindstrom, L.H., Gunne, L.M., Oest, L.G. and Person, E.: Thyrotropin-releasing hormone (TRH) in chronic schizophrenia. *Acta Psychiat. Scand.,* 55:74-80, 1977.

160. Liotta, A.S., Suda, T., and Kieger, D.T.: β-Lipotropin is the major opioid-like peptide of human and rat pars distalis: Lack of significant β-endorphin. *Proc. Nat. Acad. Sci.,* 75:2950-2954, 1978.

161. Lipton, M.A., Bissette, G., Nemeroff, C.B., Loosen, P.T., and Prange, A.J., Jr.: Neurotensin: a possible mediator of thermoregulation in the mouse. In P. Lomax and E. Schonbaum (Eds.): *Drugs, Biogenic Amines and Thermoregulation,* S. Karger, Basel, 1976.

162. Lipton, M.A., and Nemeroff, C.B.: An overview of the biogenic amine hypothesis of schizophrenia. In W.E. Fann, I. Karacan, A.D. Pokorny, and R. Williams (Eds.): *Phenomenology and Treatment of Schizophrenia,* 1977, pp. 431-454.

Psychotropic Drug Research

163. Lipton, M.A., and Goodwin, F.K.: A controlled study of thyrotropin releasing hormone in hospitalized depressed patients. *Psychopharmacol. Bull.,* 11(1):28-29, 1975.
164. Lipton, M.A., Ervin, G.N., Birkemo, L.S., Nemeroff, C.B. and Prange, A.J., Jr.: Neurotensin-neuroleptic similarities: An example of peptide-catecholamine interactions. In E. Usdin, I.J. Kopin and J. Barchas (Eds.), *Catecholamines: Basic and Clinical Frontiers,* Vol. I, Pergamon Press, N.Y., 1979, pp. 657-662.
165. Loosen, P.T., Prange, A.J., Jr., Wilson, I.C., and Lara, P.P.: Pituitary responses to thyrotropin releasing hormone in depressed patients: A review. *Pharmacol. Biochem. Behav.* (Suppl. 1), 5:95-101, 1976.
166. Loosen, P.T., Wilson, I.C., Lara, P.P., Prange, A.J., Jr., and Pettus, C.: Treatment of depressive state in alcohol withdrawal syndromes by thyrotropin releasing hormone. *Arzneimittelforschung (Drug Research),* 26:1164-1166, 1976.
167. Loosen, P.T., Nemeroff, C.B., Bissette, G., Burnett, G.B., Prange, A.J., Jr., and Lipton, M.A.: Neurotensin-induced hypothermia in the rat: Structure-activity studies. *Neuropharmacology,* 17:109-113, 1977.
168. Loosen, P.T., and Prange, A.J., Jr.: Alcohol and anterior pituitary secretion. *Lancet,* ii:985, 1977.
169. Loosen, P.T., Prange, A.J., Jr., Wilson, I.C., Lara, P.P., and Pettus, C.: Thyroid stimulating hormone response after thyrotropin releasing hormone in depressed, schizophrenic and normal women. *Psychoneuroendocrinology,* 2:137-148, 1977.
170. Loosen, P.T., Prange, A.J., Jr., and Wilson, I.C.: Influence of cortisol on TRH induced TSH response in depression. *Am. J. Psychiatry,* 135:244-246, 1978.
171. Loosen, P.T., and Prange, A.J., Jr.: The TSH response to TRH in depressed women and in depressed alcoholic men. In D. Goodwin (Ed.): *Alcohol and Affective Disorders,* Spectrum Press, Holliswood, New York, (in press).
172. Loosen, P.T., Prange, A.J., Jr., and Wilson, I.C.: TRH (Proterolin) in depressed alcoholic men: Behavioral changes and endocrine responses. *Arch. Gen. Psychiatry,* 36(5):540-547, 1979.
173. Loosen, P.T., Prange, A.J., Jr., and Wilson, I.C.: Pituitary hormone responses to TRH challenge in psychiatric patients: Their relationship to peripheral hormones. *Arch. Gen. Psychiatry,* (in press).
174. Loosen, P.T., Prange, A.J., Jr., and Wilson, I.C.: The TSH response to TRH in psychiatric patients: Relation to serum cortisol. *Prog. Neuropsychopharmacol.,* 2:479-486, 1978.
175. MacKenzie, R.G., and Trulson, M.E.: Does insulin act directly on the brain to increase tryptophan levels? *J. Neurochem.* 30:1205-1208, 1978.
176. Maeda, K., Kato, Y., Ohgo, S., Chihara, K., Yoshimoto, Y., Yamaguchi, N., Kuromaru, S., and Imura, H.: Growth hormone and pro-

lactin release after injection of thyrotropin releasing hormone in patients with depression. *J. Clin. Endocr. Metab.,* 40:501-505, 1975.

177. Maggini, C., Guazzelli M., Mauri, M., Carrara, S., Fornaro, P., Martino, E., Macchia, E., and Baschieri, L.: Sleep, clinical and endocrine studies in depressive patients treated with thyrotropin releasing hormone. In W.P. Koella, P. Levin and M. Bertini (Eds.): *Second European Congress of Sleep,* S. Karger, Basel, 1974.

178. Makino, T., Carraway, R.E., Leeman, S.E., and Greep, R.O.: *In vitro* effects of newly purified hypothalamic tridecapeptide on rat LH and FSH release. *Soc. Study Reprod.,* Abstract No. 26, 1973.

179. Malthe-Sorenssen, D., Wood, P.L., Cheney, D.L., and Costa, E.: Modulation of the turnover rate of acetylcholine in rat brain by intraventricular injections of thyrotropin-releasing hormone, somatostatin, neurotensin and angiotensin II. *J. Neurochem.,* 31:685-691, 1978.

180. Manberg, P.J., Nemeroff, C.B., and Prange, A.J., Jr.: TRH and amphetamine: A comparison of pharmacological profiles in animals. *Prog. Neuropsychopharmacol.,* (in press).

181. Martens, S., Leach, B.E., Heath, R.G., and Cohen, M.: Glutathione levels in mental and physical illness, *Arch. Neurol, Psychiatry.* 76: 630-634, 1956.

182. McAdoo, B.C., Doering, C.H., Kraemer, H.C., Dessert, N., Brodie, H.K.H., and Hamburg, D.A.: A study of the effect of gonadotropin releasing hormone on human mood and behavior. *Psychoso. Med.,* 40:199-209, 1978.

183. McCaul, J.A., Cassell, K.J., and Stern, G.M.: Intravenous thyrotropin releasing hormone in Parkinson's disease. *Lancet,* ii:735, 1974.

184. Meister, A., and Tate, S.S.: Glutathione and related f-glutamyl compounds: Biosynthesis and utilization. *Ann. Rev. Biochem.,* 45:559-603, 1976.

185. Mendelson, T.H., and Mello, N.K.: Behavioral and biochemical interactions in alcoholism. *Am. Rev. Acad.* 27: 321-333, 1976.

186. Meyer, J.H., and Grossman, M.I.: Release of secretin and cholecystokinin. In L. Demling, (Ed.): *Gastrointestinal Hormones,* Springer-Verlag, Stuttgart, 1972, p. 43.

187. Miller, L.H., Kastin, A.J., Sandman, C.A., Fink, M., and van Veen, W.J.: Polypeptide influences on attention, memory and anxiety in man. *Pharmacol. Biochem. Behav.,* 2:663-668, 1974.

188. Miller, L.H., Rischer, S.C., Groves, G.A., Rudrauff, M.E., and Kastin, A.J.: MSH/ACTH$_{4-10}$ influences on the CAR in human subjects: A negative finding. *Pharmacol. Biochem. Behav.,* 7:417-419, 1977.

189. Moldow, R.L., and Yalow, R.S.: Extrahypophyseal distribution of thyrotropin as a function of brain size. *Life Sci.,* 22:1859-1864, 1978.

190. Mortimer, C.H., McNeilly, A.S., Fisher, R.A., Murray, M.A.F., and Besser, G.M.: Gonadotropin-releasing hormone therapy in hypogonadal males with hypothalamic or pituitary dysfunction. *Br. Med. J.,* 4:617-621, 1974.

Psychotropic Drug Research

191. Moss, R.L., and McCann, S.M.: Induction of mating behavior in rats by luteinizing hormone-releasing factor. *Science*, 181:177-179, 1973.
192. Moss, R.L.: Relationship between the central regulation of gonadotropin and mating behavior in female rats. In W. Montagna and W.A. Sadler, (Eds.): *Reproductive Behavior*, Plenum Press, New York, 1975, pp. 55-76.
193. Mountjoy, C.Q., Weller, M., Hall, R., Price, J.S., Hunter, P., and Dewar, J.H.: A double-blind crossover sequential trial of oral thyrotropin-releasing hormone in depression. *Lancet*, I:958-960, 1974.
194. Mueller, K., and Hsiao, H.: Specificity of cholecystokinin satiety effect: Reduction of food but not water intake. *Pharmacol. Biochem. Behav.* 6:643-646, 1977.
195. Munn, C.: Insulin in catatonic stupor. *Arch. Neur. Psychiatry,* 34:262-269, 1935.
196. Nagai, K., and Frohman, L.A.: Hyperglycemia and Hyperglucagonemia following neurotensin administration. *Life Sci.* 19:273-280, 1976.
197. Nair, R.M.G., Kastin, A.J., and Schally, A.V.: Isolation and structure of another hypothalamic peptide possessing MSH-release inhibiting activity. *Biochem. Biophys. Res. Commun,* 47:1420-1425, 1972.
198. Nemeroff, C.B., Bissette, G., Prange, A.J., Jr., Loosen, P.T., and Lipton, M.A.: Neurotensin: central nervous system effects of a hypothalamic peptide. *Brain Res.* 128:485-496, 1977.
199. Nemeroff, C.B., Prange, A.J., Jr., Bissette, G., Loosen, P.T., Burnett, G.B., Kraemer, G.W., McKinney, W.T., and Lipton, M.A.: Effects of neurotensin on thermoregulatory processes: comparative phylogenetic studies. *Proc. Eighth Int. Conf. Psychoneuroendocrinology,* Atlanta, Ga., 1977.
200. Nemeroff, C.B., Bissette, G., Manberg, P.J., Osbahr, A.J., III, Breese, G.R., Loosen, P.T., Lipton, M.A., and Prange, A.J., Jr.: Effects of pharmacological and endocrinological manipulation on neurotensin-induced hypothermia. *Soc. Neuroscience* 4:412, 1978.
201. Nemeroff, C.B., Osbahr, A.J., III, Bissette, G., Jahnke, G., Lipton, M.A., and Prange, A.J., Jr.: Cholecystokinin inhibits tail pinch-induced eating in rats. *Science,* 200:793-794, 1978.
202. Nemeroff, C.B., and Prange, A.J., Jr.: Peptides and psychoneuroendochrinology, A perspective. *Arch. Gen. Psychiatry*, 35:999-1010, 1978.
203. Nemeroff, C.B., Loosen, P.T., Bissette, G., Manberg, P.J., Lipton, M.A., and Prange, A.J., Jr.: Pharmaco-behavioral effects of hypothalamic peptides in animals and man: Focus on thyrotropin-releasing hormone and neurotensin. *Psychoneuroendocrinology,* (in press).
204. Nemeroff, C.B., Osbahr, A.J., III, Ervin, G.N., and Prange, A.J., Jr.: Evaluation of the analgesic effect of centrally administered neuropeptides. *Am. Soc. Neurochem.,* 10th Annual meeting, Charleston, S.C. abstract (in press).
205. Obiols, J., Pujol, J., and Obiols-Llandrich, J.: Hormonas hipotalamicas

Peptides in Mental Disorders

y function tiroidea en los sindromes de presivos. Presented at *1st World Congress of Biological Psychiatry,* Buenos Aires, September, 1974.

206. Orci, L., Baetens, O., Rufener, C., Brown, M., Vale, W., and Guillemin, R.: Evidence for immunoreactive neurotensin in dog intestinal mucosa. *Life Sci.* 19:559-562, 1977.

207. Ormston, B.J., Garry, R., Cryer, R.J., Besser, G.M., and Hall, R.: TRH as a thyroid function test. *Lancet,* ii:10, 1971.

208. Osbahr, A.J., III, Nemeroff, C.B., Manberg, P.J., and Prange, A.J., Jr.: Centrally administered neurotensin: Activity in the Julou-Courvoisier muscle relaxation test in mice. *Eur. J. Pharmacol.* 54:299-302, 1979.

209. Pagano, R.R., and Lovely, R.H.: Diurnal cycle and ACTH facilitation of shuttle-box avoidance. *Physiol. Behav.* 8:721-723, 1972.

210. Pearse, A.G.G.: Diffuse neuroendocrine peptides common to brain and intestine and their relationship to the APUD concept. In J. Hughes, (Ed.): *Centrally Acting Peptides,* MacMillan Press, London, 1978, pp. 49-57.

211. Pecknold, L.C., and Ban, T.A.: TRH in depressive illness. *Pharmacopsychiatry,* 12:166-173, 1977.

212. Pijnenberg, A.J.J., Honig, W.M.M., and van Rossum, J.M.: Effects of antagonists upon locomotor stimulation induced by injection of dopamine and noradrenaline into the nucleus accumbens of the rat. *Psychopharmacologia* (Berl.), 41:87-95, 1975.

213. Pijneberg, A.J.J., Honig, W.M.M., and van Rossum, J.M.: Inhibition of d-amphetamine-induced locomotor activity by injection of haloperidol into the nucleus accumbens of the rat. *Psychopharmacologia (Berl.),* 41:87-95, 1975.

214. Plotnikoff, N.P., Kastin, A.J., Anderson, M.S., and Schally, A.V.: DOPA potentiation by a hypothalamic factor, MSH release-inhibiting hormone (MIF). *Life Sci.,* 10:1279-1283, 1971.

215. Plotnikoff, N.P., Prange, A.J., Jr., Breese, G.R., Anderson, M.S., and Wilson, I.C.: Thyrotropin releasing hormone: enhancement of DOPA activity by a hypothalamic hormone. *Science,* 178:417-418, 1972.

216. Plotnikoff, N.P., Prange, A.J., Jr., Breese, G.R., Anderson, M.S., and Wilson, I.C.: The effects of thyrotropin-releasing hormone on DOPA response in normal, hypophysectomized and thyroidectomized animals. In A.J. Prange, Jr., (Ed.): *The Thyroid Axis, Drugs, and Behavior,* Raven Press, New York, 1974, pp. 103-114.

217. Popovic, V., and Popovic, P.: *Hypothermia in Biology and Medicine.* Grune and Stratton, New York, 1974.

218. Prange, A.J., Jr., Wilson, I.C., Rabon, A.M., and Lipton, M.A.: Enhancement of imipramine antidepressant activity by thyroid hormone. *Am. J. Psychiatry,* 126:457-469, 1969.

219. Prange, A.J., Jr., Wilson, I.C., Knox, A., McClane, T.K., and Lipton, M.A.: Enhancement of imipramine by thyroid stimulating hormone:

Psychotropic Drug Research

Clinical and theoretical implications. *Am. J. Psychiatry,* 127(2):191-199, 1970.

220. Prange, A.J., Jr., and Wilson, I.C.: Thyrotropin releasing hormone (TRH) for the immediate relief of depression: A preliminary report. *Psychopharmacologia.* 26:82, 1972.

221. Prange, A.J., Jr., Wilson, I.C., Lara, P.P., Alltop, L.B., and Breese, G.R.: Effects of thyrotropin-releasing hormone in depression. *Lancet,* ii:999-1002, 1972.

222. Prange, A.J., Jr., Wilson, I.C., Lynn, C.W., Alltop, L.B., and Stikelether, R.A.: L-tryptophan in mania: Contribution to a permissive hypothesis of affective disorders. *Arch. Gen. Psychiatry,* 5:56-62, 1974.

223. Prange, A.J., Jr., Wilson, I.C., Breese, G.R., and Lipton, M.A.: Behavioral effects of hypothalamic releasing hormones in animals and man. In W.H. Gispen, T.B. van Wimersma Greidanus, B. Bohus and D. de Wied, (Eds.): *Hormones, Homeostasis and the Brain, Progress in Brain Research,* Vol. 42, Elsevier, Amsterdam, 1975, pp. 1-9.

224. Prange, A.J., Jr.: Patterns of pituitary responses to thyrotropin releasing hormone in depressed patients: A review. In W.E. Fann, I. Karacan, A. Pokorny and R.L. Williams (Eds.): *Phenomenology and Treatment of Depression,* Spectrum Publishing Company, New York, 1976, pp. 1-15.

225. Prange, A.J., Jr., Breese, G.R., Wilson, I.C., and Lipton, M.A.: Brain-behavioral effects of hypothalamic releasing hormones: A generic hypothesis. In W.E. Stumpf and L.D. Grant, (Eds.): *Anatomical Neuroendocrinology,* S. Karger, Basel, 1976, pp. 357-367.

226. Prange, A.J., Jr., Lipton, M.A., Nemeroff, C.B., and Wilson, I.C.: The role of hormones in depression. *Life Sci.,* 20:1305-1318, 1977.

227. Prange, A.J., Jr., Nemeroff, C.B., and Lipton, M.A.: Behavioral effects of peptides: Basic and clinical studies. In M.A. Lipton, A. DiMascio, and K.F. Killam (Eds.): *Psychopharmacology: A Generation of Progress,* Raven Press, New York, 1978, pp. 441-458.

228. Prange, A.J., Jr., Nemeroff, C.B., Lipton, M.A., Breese, G.R., and Wilson, I.C.: Peptides and the central nervous system. In L.L. Iversen, S.D. Iversen and S.H. Snyder (Eds.): *Handbook of Psychopharmacology,* Vol. 13, Plenum Publishing, New York, 1978, pp. 1-107.

229. Prange, A.J., Jr., Nemeroff, C.B., and Loosen, P.T.: Behavioral effects of hypothalamic peptides. In J. Hughes (Ed.): *Centrally Acting Peptides,* The MacMillan Press Ltd., Basingstoke, England, 1978, pp. 99-118.

230. Puca, A.: La insulino-terapia nei malati di mente. *Rass. Studi, Psichiat.* 16:461, 1927.

231. Rafaelsen, O.J., and Mellerup, E.: Insulin action. In A. Lajtha, (Ed.): *Handbook of Neurochemistry,* Vol. IV, Plenum Press, New York, 1970, pp. 361-371.

232. Rapoport, J.L., Quinn, P.Q., Copeland, A.P., and Burg, C.:

ACTH$_{4-10}$: Cognitive and behavioral effects in hyperactive, learning disabled children. *Neuropsychobiology,* 2:291-296, 1976.

233. Redmond, G.P., Bell, J.J., and Perel, J.M.: Effect of human growth hormone on amobarbital metabolism in children. *Clin. Pharmacol. Ther.,* 24:213-218, 1978.

234. Rehfeld, J.F., and Kruse-Larsen, C.: Gastrin and cholecystokinin in human cerebrospinal fluid. Immunochemical determination of concentrations and molecular heterogeneity. *Brain Res.,* 155:19-26, 1978.

235. Rigter, H., van Riezen, H., and deWied, D.: The effects of ACTH and vasopressin-analogues on CO_2-induced retrograde amnesia in rats. *Physiol. Behav.,* 13:381-388, 1974.

236. Rigter, H., Elbertse, R., and van Riezen, H.: Time-dependent antiamnesic effect of ACTH and desglycinamidelysine vasopressin. In W.H. Gispen, T. B. van Wimersma Greidanus and B. Bohus, et al., (Eds.): *Hormones, Homeostasis and the Brain,* Amsterdam, Elsevier, 1975.

237. Rinkel, M., and Hirmuich, H.E.: *Insulin Treatment in Psychiatry,* Philosophical Library, New York, 1959.

238. Rivier, C., Brown, M., and Vale, W.: Effect of neurotensin, substance P, and morphine sulfate on the secretion of prolactin and growth hormone in the rat. *Endocrinology,* 100:751-754.

239. Rivier, J.E., Lazarus, L.H., Perrin, M.H., and Brown, M.R.: Neurotensin analogues: Structure-activity relationships. *J. Med. Chem.,* 20:1409-1412, 1977.

240. Sakel, M.: *Neur Behandlungsmethode der Schizophrenie,* Vienna: Verlag Moritz Perles, 1935.

241. Sandman, C.A., George, J., Walker, B.B., and Nolan, J.D.: Neurotetrapeptide MSH/ACTH$_{4-10}$ enhances attention in the mentally retarded. *Pharmacol. Biochem. Behav.,* 5: Suppl. 1, 23-28, 1976.

242. Sandman, C.A., George, J., McCanne, R.T., Nolan, J.D., Kasman, J., and Kastin, A.J.: MSH/ACTH$_{4-10}$ influences behavioral and physiological measures of attention. *J. Clin. Endo. Metab.,* 44:884-891, 1977.

243. Sannita, W.G., Irwin, P., and Fink, M.: EEG and task performances after ACTH$_{4-10}$ in man. *Neuropsychobiology,* 2:283-290, 1976.

244. Sarne, Y., Azov, R., and Weissman, B.A.: A stable enkephalin-like immunoreactive substance in human CSF. *Brain Res.,* 151:399-403, 1978.

245. Sawin, C.T., and Hershman, J.M.: Clinical use of thyrotropin-releasing hormone. *Clin. Pharmacol. Ther.,* 1:351-366, 1976.

246. Schally, A.V.: Aspects to hypothalamic regulation of the pituitary gland. *Science,* 202:18-28, 1978.

247. Schmidt, P.: Uber organtherapie und insulinbehandlung bei endogenen geistesstorungen. *Klin. Woch.,* 7:839, 1928.

248. Schneider, A.M., Weinberg, J., and Weissberg, R.: Effects of ACTH on conditioned suppression: A time and strength of conditioning analysis. *Physiol. Behav.,* 13:633-636, 1974.

249. Shopsin, B., Shenkman, L., Blum, M., and Hollander, C.: T₃ and TSH response to TRH: Newer aspects of lithium-induced thyroid disturbances in men. *Psychopharm. Bull.,* 9:29, 1973.

250. Sicuteri, F., Anselmi, B., Curradi, C., Midraelacci, S., and Sassi, A.: Morphine-like factors in CSF of headache patients. In E. Costa and M. Trabucchi, (Eds.): *The Endorphins,* Raven Press, New York, 1978.

251. Siler, T.M., Van den Berg, G., and Yen, S.S.C.: Inhibition of growth hormone release in human by somatostatin. *J. Clin. Endocrinol. Metab.,* 37:632-634, 1973.

252. Sjolund, B., Terenius, L., and Eriksson, M.: Increased cerebrospinal fluid levels of endorphins after electro-acupuncture. *Acta Physiol. Scand.,* 100:283-384, 1977.

253. Slotopolsky, B.: Insulin bei nahrungsverweigernden geisteskranken. *Z. Neur. Psych.,* 136:367, 1931.

254. Snyder, P.J., and Utiger, R.D.: Response to thyrotropin releasing hormone in normal man. *J. Clin. Endocrinol. Metab.,* 34:380, 1972.

255. Snyder, P.J., and Utiger, R.D.: Thyrotropin response to thyrotropin releasing hormone in normal females over forty. *J. Clin. Endocrinol. Metab.,* 34:1096, 1972.

256. Snyder, S.H.: Amphetamine psychosis: A "model" schizophrenia mediated by catecholamines. *Am. J. Psychiatry,* 130:61-67, 1973.

257. Smith, G.P., and Gibbs, J.: Cholecystokinin: A putative satiety signal, *Pharmacol. Biochem. Behav.,* 3 (Suppl. 1): 135-138, 1975.

258. Smith, G.P., and Gibbs, J.: Cholecystokinin and satiety: Theoretic and therapeutic implications. In D. Novin, G.A. Bray and W. Wyrwicka, (Eds.): *Hunger: Basic Mechanism and Clinical Implications,* Raven Press, New York, 1975, pp.19-29.

259. Smith, G.P., and Cushin, B.J.: Cholecystokinin acts at a vagally innervated abdominal site to elicit satiety. *Soc. Neuroscience Abstracts,* 4:180, 1978.

260. Sorensen, R., Svendsen, K., and Schou, M.: TRH in depression. *Lancet,* ii:865-866, 1974.

261. Stokes, P.E.: Alcohol-endocrine interrelationships. In B. Kissin, and H. Begleiter, (Eds.): *The Biology of Alcoholism,* Plenum Press, New York, 1971, Vol. I, pp. 397-436.

262. Strand, F.L., Cayer, A., Gonzalez, E., and Stoboy, H.: Peptide enhancement of neuromuscular function: animal and clinical studies. *Pharmacol. Biochem. Behav.* 5: Suppl. 1, 179-187, 1976.

263. Straus, E., and Yalow, R.S.: Species specificity of cholecystokinin in gut and brain of several mammalian species. *Proc. Natl. Acad. Sci.,* 75:486-489, 1978.

264. Sturdevant, R.A.L., and Goetz, H.: Cholecystokinin both stimulates and inhibits human food intake. *Nature,* 261:714-715, 1976.

265. Sugarman, A.A., Mueller, P.S., Swartzburg, M., and Rockford, J.: Abbott-38579 (Synthetic TRH) in the treatment of depression: A

controlled study of oral administration. *Psychopharmacol. Bull.* 11 (1):30, 1975.

266. Tagliamonte, A., DeMontis, M.G., Olianas, M., Onali, P.L., and Gessa, G.L.: Possible role of insulin in the transport of tyrosine and tryptophan from blood to brain. *Pharmac. Res. Commun.,* 7:493-499, 1975.

267. Takahashi, S., Kondo, H., Yoshimura, M., and Ochi, Y.: Thyrotropin responses to TRH in depressive illness: Relation to clinical subtypes and prolonged duration of depressive episode. *Folia Psychiat. Neurol. Jpn.,* 28:355-365, 1974.

268. Tamminga, C.A., Schaffer, M.H., Smith, R.C., and Davis, J.M.: Schizophrenic symptoms improve with apomorphine. *Science,* 200:567-568, 1978.

269. Targowla, R., and Lamache, A.: Le traitement pal l'insuline des états d'anorexie de sitiophobie et de dénutrition dans les troubles psychonévropathiques. *Prat. Med. Franc.,* 5:452, 1926.

270. Terenius, L., Wahlstrom, A., and Agren, A.: Naloxone (Narcan) treatment in depression: Clinical observations and effects on CSF endorphin and macroamino metabolites. *Psychopharmacology,* 54:31-33, 1977.

271. Terenius, L., and Wahlstrom, A.: Physiological and clinical relevance of endorphins. In J. Hughes (Ed.): *Centrally Acting Peptides,* MacMillan Press, Ltd., London, 1978, pp. 161-178.

272. van Thiel, D.H. and Lester, R.: Alcoholism: Its effects on hypothalamic-pituitary-gonadal function. *Gastroenterology,* 71:318-327, 1976.

273. Tiwary, G.M., Rosenbloom, A.L., Robertson, M.F., and Parker, J.C.: Effects of thyrotropin releasing hormone in minimal brain dysfunction. *Pediatrics,* 56(1):119-121, 1975.

274. Torjesen, P.A., Haug, E., and Sand, T.: Effect of TRH on serum levels of pituitary hormones in men and women. *Acta Endocrinol.* (kbh) 73: 455, 1973.

275. Tsuang, M.T., and Winokur, G.: Criteria for subtyping schizophrenia, *Arch. Gen. Psychiatry,* 31:43-47, 1974.

276. Turek, I.S., and Rocha, J.: Oral thyrotropin-releasing hormone (TRH) in depressive illness. *J. Clin. Pharmacol.* 14:612-616, 1974.

277. Uhl, G.R., Bennett, J.P., Jr., and Snyder, S.H.: Neurotensin, a central nervous system peptide: Apparent receptor binding in brain membranes. *Brain Res.,* 130:299-313, 1977.

278. Uhl, G.R., Kuhar, M.J., and Snyder, S.H.: Neurotensin: Immunohistochemical localization in rat central nervous system. *Proc. Natl. Acad. Sci.,* 74:4059-4063, 1977.

279. Uhl, G.R., and Snyder, S.H.: Regional and subcellular distribution of brain neurotensin. *Life Sci.,* 19:1827-1832, 1977.

280. Van den Burg, W., van Praag, H.M., Bos, E.R.H., Piers, D.A., van Zanton, A.K., and Doorenbos, H.: TRH as a possible quick-acting but short-lasting antidepressant. *Psychol. Med.,* 5:404-412, 1975.

Psychotropic Drug Research

281. Van den Burg, W., van Praag, H.M., Bos, E.R.H. Piers, D.A., van Zanton, A.K., and Doorenbos, H.: TRH by slow, continuous infusion: An antidepressant? *Psychol. Med.,* 6:393-397, 1976.

282. Van der Vis-Melsen, M.J.E., and Wiener, J.D.: Improvement in mental depression with decreased thyrotropin response after administration of thyrotropin-releasing hormone. *Lancet,* ii:1415, 1972.

283. van Riezen, H., Rigter, H., and de Wied, D.: Possible significance of ACTH fragments for human mental performance. *Behav. Biol.,* 20: 311-324, 1977.

284. van Wimersma Greidanus, T.B., Dogterom J., and de Wied, D.: Intraventricular administration of antivasopressin serum inhibits memory consolidation in rats. *Life Sci.,* 16:637-644, 1975.

285. Vanamee, P., Winawer, S.J., Sherlock, P., Sonnenberg, M., and Lipkin, M.: Decreased incidence of restraint-stress induced gastric erosions in rats treated with bovine growth hormone. *Proc. Soc. Exp. Biol. Med.,* 135:259-262, 1970.

286. Verebey, K., Volavka, J., and Clovet, D.: Endorphins in psychiatry. *Arch. Gen. Psychiatry,* 35:877-888, 1978.

287. Verhoeven, W.M.A., van Praag, H.M., Botter, P.A., Souncer, A., van Ree, J.M., and de Wied, D.: (Des-Tyr[1])-γ-endorphin in schizophrenia. *Lancet,* i:1046-1047, 1978.

288. Vogel, H.P., Benkert, O., Illig, R., Mueller-Oerlinghausen, B., and Poppenberg, A.: Psychoendocrinological and therapeutic effects of TRH in depression. *Acta Psychiat. Scand.,* 56:223-232, 1977.

289. Volavka, J., Mallya, A., Baig, S., and Perez-Cruet, J.: Naloxone in chronic schizophrenia. *Science,* 196:1227-1228, 1977.

290. von Graffenreid, B., del Pozo, E., Roubicek, J., Krebs, E., Poldinger, W., Burmeister, P., and Kerp, L.: Effects of the synthetic enkephalin analogue FK33-824 in man. *Nature,* 272:729-730, 1978.

291. Walter, R., Hoffman, P.L., and Flexner, J.B.: Neurophypophyseal hormones, analogs, and fragments: Their effects on puromycin-induced amnesia. *Proc. Natl. Acad. Sci. U.S.A.,* 72:4180-4183, 1975.

292. Watson, S.J., Berger, P.A., Akil, H., Mills, M.J., and Barchas, J.D.: Effect of naloxone on schizophrenia: Reduction in hallucinations in a subpopulation of subjects. *Science,* 201:73-76, 1978.

293. Weeke, A., and Weeke, J.: Disturbed circadian variation of serum thyrotropin in patients with endogenous depression. *Acta. Psychiatry Scand.,* 57:281-289, 1978.

294. Wenzel, K.W., Meinhold, A., Herpich, M., Adlkofer, F., and Schleusener, H.: TRH stimulationstest mit alters - und geschlechtsabhaengigem TSH - Anstieg bei normalpersonen. *Klin. Wschr.,* 52:722-727, 1974.

295. Widerlov, E., and Sjostrom, R.: Effects of thyrotropin releasing hormone on endogenous depression. *Nord. Psychiat. T.,* 29:503-512, 1975.

296. Wilson, I.C., Prange, A.J., Jr., McClane, T.K., Rabon, A.M., and Lipton, M.A.: Thyroid hormone enhancement of imipramine in non-

retarded depression. *N. Eng. J. Med.,* 282:1063-1067, 1970.

297. Wilson, I.C., Lara, P.P., and Prange, A.J., Jr.: Thyrotropin releasing hormone in schizophrenia. *Lancet,* ii:43-44, 1973.

298. Wilson, I.C., Prange, A.J., Jr., Lara, P.P., Alltop, L.B., Stikeleather, R.A., and Lipton, M.A.: TRH (lopremone): Psychobiological responses of normal women: (I) subjective experience. *Arch. Gen. Psychiatry,* 29:15-32, 1973.

299. Winawer, S.J., Sherlock, P., Sonnenberg, M., and Vanamee, P.: Beneficial effect of human growth hormone on stress ulcers. *Arch. Intern. Med.,* 135:569-572, 1975.

300. Winokur, A., and Utiger, R.D.:Thyrotropin-releasing hormone: Regional distribution in rat brain. *Science,* 185:265-266, 1974.

301. Winokur, G., Cadoret, R., Dorzab, T., and Baker, M.: Depressive disease, a genetic study. *Arch. Gen. Psychiatry,* 24:135-144, 1971.

302. Ylikahri, R.H., Huttunen, M.O., and Harkonen, M.: Effect of alcohol on anterior pituitary secretion of trophic hormones. *Lancet.* i:1353, 1976.

303. Youngblood, W.E., Lipton, M.A., and Kizer, J.S.: TRH-like immunoreactivity in urine, serum and extra-hypothalamic brain: Non-identity with synthetic pyroglu-his-pro-NH$_2$ (TRH). *Brain Res.,* 151: 99-116, 1978.

7

The Effects of Drugs in Episodic Dyscontrol Disorders

GEORGE U. BALIS, M.D.

I. INTRODUCTION

The objective of this paper is to present a brief review of current concepts regarding the so-called "Episodic Dyscontrol Disorders," as a basis for formulating working hypotheses which could assist in developing approaches to the diagnostic differentiation and treatment of these disorders.

II. REVIEW OF THE CONCEPT OF EPISODIC DYSCONTROL DISORDERS

A number of investigators have contributed to the recognition of this syndrome, including Karl Menninger (38), Russell Monroe (41), Ervin (34), and others (5, 31, 45). This clinical work has converged towards an effort to define the syndrome as a discrete diagnostic entity. As a matter of fact, the forthcoming DSM III has incorporated this nosologic concept into a new diagnostic category labelled "Intermittent Explosive Disorder" which is classified under the Axis II heading "Disorders of Impulse Control." It is noted that many of the patients belonging to this category were previously diagnosed, under the DSM II, as "Explosive Personality." Other terms used in the literature to describe this group of patients include "Episodic Behavioral Disorders" and "Limbic System Disorder."

A. Etiology

Although it is generally recognized that there is a complex inter-

George U. Balis, M.D. is Professor at the Institute of Psychiatry and Human Behavior, University of Maryland Medical School, Baltimore, Maryland.

Psychotropic Drug Research

action between neurophysiological and psychological factors in contributing to the development of the syndrome, most authors postulate the presence of an underlying neurophysiological dysfunction. Presumptive evidence for this brain dysfunction is based on the frequent occurrence of "soft" neurological signs which are suggestive of an "epileptoid" origin associated with "organicity." The paroxysmal criterion that characterizes the episodic occurrence of these disorders has been the most significant differentiating clinical feature and has been used as evidence to support the presumed epileptic nature of the brain dysfunction. However, the absence of sufficient evidence of specific paroxysmal electroencephalographic (EEG) abnormalities has been a major argument against an epileptic mechanism. On the other hand, it has been argued that a normal EEG does not preclude the possibility of an underlying epileptic etiology. This is based on the observation that the routine scalp EEG may be normal in known epileptics, and that repeated serial EEGs markedly increase the incidence of positive findings. Also, data from implanted electrodes studies show that excessive neuronal discharges can occur in subcortical areas without any reflection in the routine scalp recordings. It is thus reasoned that the postulated brain dysfunction may be associated with limited ictal discharges in subcortical structures, and that such discharges may be accompanied by behavioral changes, not usually identified as epileptic. More specifically, Mark and Ervin (34) suggest that the dysfunction represents a focal ictal disorder of the limbic system, and stress the apparent similarities between the syndrome and temporal lobe epilepsy. Some postulate that "subictal" electrical discharges in the limbic structures, and especially the amygdala, may exercise a "kindling effect" that results in the lowering of the seizural threshold (29). Mark (35) attributes the longer duration of the behavior dyscontrol disorders to "long latency effects," that is, behavioral changes resulting from brain stimulation that outlasts after-discharges. He proposes that these disorders, while not truly ictal, result from a previous ictus (postictal).

Since aggressive-violent behavior of an explosively episodic character is considered to be an essential feature of the syndrome, there has been great effort to relate the brain dysfunction underlying the syndrome to mechanisms associated with the modulation of aggression. Drawing from a large amount of neurophysiological and clinical studies, various authors have attempted to associate violence with hypothalamic involvement (1, 24, 51) or with lesions in the limbic system (34), and by analogy, to attribute the etiology of

192

the episodic dyscontrol disorders to disturbances localized in the same brain structures. Nevertheless, the proposed limbic localization of violent behavior continues to be controversial (66). Furthermore, in our experience, it appears that although outbursts of violence is a very common and striking feature of the syndrome, it may not be an essential one, and that, therefore, the definition of the syndrome in the DSM III as "Intermittent Explosive Disorder" may be unduly restrictive.

In the effort to provide evidence supporting the postulated epileptic etiology of the syndrome, many authors have stressed its apparent similarity with certain ictal, postictal, and interictal manifestations of the temporal lobe epilepsy, and especially with regard to the alleged high incidence of aggressive-violent behavior in the latter condition. Paroxysmal outbursts or irritability, anger, aggressive impulses, and rage, have been reported to be frequent ictal manifestations of temporal lobe epilepsy, occurring in clear consciousness or with varying degrees of amnesia of the episode. Aggressive acts of consummatory nature may also occur during ictal twilight states and may range from episodes of violent behavior to attack or even homicide. Furthermore, postictal episodes may begin or be followed by a period of delirious excitement lasting for several minutes or hours, and in some instances for days or weeks. This delirious-like state may consist, at times, of dramatic outbursts of agitation associated with paranoid ideation and hallucinations and may lead to repetitive acts of extremely violent aggression, and occasionally murder. The aggressive acts committed during such prolonged postictal episodes are characteristically violent and brutal, as compared to aggressive acts committed during a psychomotor attack. During the postictal episode, the patient shows altered consciousness, appears to be confused and disoriented, and presents complete amnesia or spotty recollection of the events surrounding the confusional period. Throughout this period, the EEG shows diffuse symmetrical slow-wave activity or a rather ill-defined low-voltage activity, with no categorical abnormalities and with notable absence of spikes (6).

Among the interictally occurring disturbances, the so-called temporal lobe epileptic personality has been described by a number of authors as constituting what is commonly known as the epileptic personality. This includes the retarded, enechetic, or viscous type, which is the most commonly encountered, as well as the explosive, aggressive or irritable type. The latter personality type shows irritability, aggressiveness, impulsivity, emotional instability, and explosiveness, with a proneness to sudden changes in mood and violent rage reactions (6). Falconer (14) has shown that interictal aggressive behavior can be eliminated by unilateral temporal lobectomy in more than 50% of the patients suffering from temporal lobe dysfunction secondary to mesial temporal lobe sclerosis. This syndrome is thought to be characterized primarily by ictal episodes of rage (6).

Many EEG studies have attempted to correlate violent or aggressive behavior with temporal lobe abnormalities. Most of these studies were conducted on prisoners, often charged with murder and known psychopaths. Several other studies, however, have failed to substantiate these findings. Similarly, several other studies have failed to confirm the reported high incidence of violent behavior in temporal lobe epileptic patients (6).

Besides violent-aggressive behavior, a number of other episodically occurring disturbances—affective, cognitive, autonomic, perceptual—have been reported to characterize patients with temporal lobe epilepsy. The same disturbances have been reported by some authors to occur in patients with episodic dyscontrol disorders. Ictal affective symptoms of depression or mania appearing during the course of temporal lobe seizures (psychic attacks) are very common. Acute feelings of despair and depression during the attack may be accompanied by suicidal impulses; in a typical attack these symptoms last for a few minutes at most. Auras of premonition of death, end of the world, or other catastrophic expectations have also been reported. In general, patients with temporal lobe EEG abnormalities with or without the presence of seizures, are frequently subject to variations of mood (depression, elation, euphoria, ecstasy, suspiciousness, irritability, hostility), often with concomitant anxiety, occurring with normal consciousness, that are not ordinarily thought to be ictal. Characteristically, the epileptic mood is of extreme sudden onset and builds up to the full extent within a few hours. The paroxysmal character of the episode (acute onset and equally acute remission, lasting for relatively short periods, and very often associated with intense anxiety) point to an ictal mechanism. A number of epileptic patients often experience mounting irritability, tension, anxiety, and depression, in spite of the fact that their seizures are well controlled under medication. These symptoms invariably subside after the patient experiences a seizure of the grand mal type. It is generally agreed that patients with temporal lobe epilepsy are particularly prone to experiencing affective disturbances, and particularly irritability and depression;

Episodic Dyscontrol Disorders

brief episodes of depressive or manic behavior which occur recurrently with a paroxysmal character in subjects who are not known to suffer from epileptic seizures may have an ictal etiology (6).

Perceptive and apperceptive disturbances, occurring as auras or during psychomotor attacks, are manifested as hallucinatory or illusory phenomena, which are generally ego-alien and are experienced and recalled as long as memory processes are not compromised by the ictal discharges (dysmnesia). Such symptoms are believed to be seldom reported by patients with episodic dyscontrol (6).

Confusional psychotic episodes of short duration are most frequent in centrencephalic epileptics, and are thought to be postictal in origin. On the other hand, schizophrenic-like psychoses are thought to be particularly frequent in patients with temporal lobe epilepsy. Numerous studies have given support to the observation that temporal lobe epileptics are characteristically prone to developing schizoid personality traits, and in some instances, schizophreniform psychoses of a paranoid type, both acute and chronic. The acute episodes usually last days or weeks, and are rarely preceded by a grand mal seizure but often end in one. During these episodes, the EEG rhythms are either normal or desynchronized with disappearance of pathological rhythms, a phenomenon referred to as "forced normalization." This reported inverse relationship between the occurrence of seizures and psychotic episodes may lead to a seesaw-like pattern. The etiology and pathogenesis of these psychotic episodes remain obscure. In the continuing controversy over the nature of the underlying mechanisms, various hypotheses have been proposed, spanning the range of both psychological and neurophysiological theorizing. Several authors have reported similar psychotic episodes occurring in non-epileptic patients with evidence of an "epileptoid" brain dysfunction, which is thought to constitute part of the episodic behavior disorders (6).

Several recent studies have suggested that there are differences in the type of behavior disorders depending on the lateralization of the epileptogenic focus. Aggressive behavior in temporal lobe epileptics has been linked with dominant hemisphere involvement and hence with speech and memory impairment. Similarly, the epileptic involvement of the dominant temporal lobe is more likely to be associated with schizophrenic-like psychosis, whereas the involvement of the nondominant temporal lobe is more likely to be associated with manic-depressive disturbances (6).

Nonepisodic psychopathology characterizing patients with tem-

195

Psychotropic Drug Research

poral lobe epilepsy, includes, in addition to the so-called "epileptic personality," frequent hypochondriacal complaints, and sexual dysfunctions, particularly hyposexuality, and in some cases, various paraphilias. "Soft" neurological signs suggestive of brain "organicity" have been reported by a number of authors. Patients with post-traumatic brain syndrome may show lability of affect, irritability, impulsivity, loss of creativity, concrete thinking, distractibility, and limited attention span, egocentricity, perseveration, and circumstantiality, organic orderliness, diminished spontaneity in thought, depressed mood changes, a tendency to paranoid suspicion, and frequent intolerance of alcohol. Furthermore, organic syndromes involving the temporal lobes are associated with similar disturbances. Also, patients with bilateral temporal lobe involvement show recent memory deficit. Patients with episodic dyscontrol disorders are also thought to show presumptive evidence of CNS "organicity" in the form of "soft" neurological signs (e.g., history of perinatal "insult" or brain injury, and deficit in higher cortical functions) (6).

Finally, several authors have postulated that episodic dyscontrol disorders are an adult expression of the "minimal brain dysfunction" (MBD), or hyperkinetic syndrome in childhood. Similarities shared by both syndromes include, history of perinatal and early childhood CNS traumata, episodically occurring symptomatology, evidence of learning difficulties, soft neurological signs, and the predominance of males. Thus, in a study of 130 violent patients with episodic dyscontrol, Bach-y-Rita (5) reported the following identifying criteria, in addition to soft neurological signs, and abnormal EEG: childhood history of hyperactivity, fighting, temper tantrums, enuresis, and nail biting. Morrison (45) refers to the "explosive personality" as a sequel of the hyperactive child syndrome; his patients had a history of childhood hyperactivity and decreased ability to concentrate. He suggests that as the hyperactivity decreases with developmental maturation it is replaced by aggressiveness and hair-trigger temper with the individual showing destructive impulsive behavior. Other retrospective studies suggest that subjects who had characteristics of the MBD syndrome in childhood, may show a variety of neurotic and characterological problems as young adults (20, 50) as well as episodic impulse dyscontrol disorders (5, 32, 68). Some suggest that the adult with a history of MBD in childhood would often show diffuse symptoms related to depression and anxiety, often without impulsiveness and hyperactivity. Important in making the diagnosis of "Adult Brain

Episodic Dyscontrol Disorders

Dysfunction" (ABD) is a family history of learning disorders, poor impulse control, alcoholism, and periodic endogenous depression (32). Few prospective studies (36, 37) of children with childhood MBD have reported the development of serious psychopathology during adolescence and early adulthood including psychosis, delinquency, and behavior described as hyperactive, impulsive, rebellious, destructive, associated with temper tantrums, and antisocial. In Menkes' study (37) of the 11 in his group of patients examined neurologically 8 had "definite evidence of neurological dysfunction," usually consisting of terminal intention tremor and minimal uncoordination. Although MBD was initially thought to represent a developmental lag, investigators have proposed many other causes, including perinatal trauma, head injury, encephalitis, poisoning (especially lead), and hereditary predisposion (28, 61, 67). More recent biological approaches have attempted to define the syndrome as resulting from a defect in amine metabolism (67). Family studies of hyperactive children suggest that 10 to 38% of the parents of these children had been hyperactive in childhood, and that those with such history show prominent symptoms of alcoholism (9).

In our experience, there seems to be a significant correlation between episodic dyscontrol disorders and Borderline Personality organization, an observation that is further supported by comparing the essential features of these poorly defined conditions. According to the DSM III, the salient features of the Unstable Personality Disorder (Borderline Personality), include: a) impulsivity or unpredictability in at least two areas which are potentially self-damaging, e.g., sex, drug or alcohol abuse, physically self-damaging acts, etc.; b) inappropriate intense anger or lack of control of anger; c) affective instability, with marked shifts from normal mood to depression, irritability or anxiety, usually lasting hours, with a return to normal mood; d) physically self-damaging acts, such as suicidal gestures, self-mutilation, recurrent accidents or physical fights; also patterns of unstable and intense interpersonal relationships, identity disturbances, problems tolerating being alone, and chronic feelings of emptiness or boredom. There is strong suggestive evidence that MBD, Unstable Personality Disorder and Episodic Dyscontrol may represent a triadic syndrome sharing, to some measure, common etiologic determinants.

In conclusion, most of the authors postulate that an essential etiological condition underlying the episodic dyscontrol disorders is a CNS dysfunction, whose nature is thought to be epileptic or "epileptoid," with a localization in the subcortical areas, and par-

197

ticularly in the temporolimbic regions, and which is associated with soft neurological signs suggestive of some "organic" brain deficit. Furthermore, there is some evidence that patients displaying this syndrome frequently report a history of minimal brain dysfunction in childhood, thus implying a common pathogenetic mechanism. The assertion that this group of disorders represents an "epileptoid" category remains problematical, in spite of the clinical similarities between epileptic disorders and episodic dyscontrol. The term "epileptoid" has been variously used to describe borderline cases, atypical forms of conventional epileptic seizures, or new provisional forms which do not strictly meet the standard criteria for the definition of epilepsy. The term introduces ambiguity and easily invites controversy, especially if one interprets it to mean an epileptic-like condition. Similarities to epileptic conditions may refer to different characteristics of variable significance, or analogous phenomena whose resemblance to epilepsy may be more apparent than real. The basic question is whether a disorder described as "epileptoid" is really epileptic in nature or only epileptic-like. It is clear that the term epileptoid can only be of some usefulness if it denotes an actually epileptic mechanism; in that sense, its use might refer to a provisional or inferred diagnosis of epilepsy in a disorder which still remains obscure. Unfortunately, some authors, who define the etiology of the syndrome as "epileptoid," make interchangeable references to both ictal mechanisms and "maturational lag" or "CNS instability" as being ismorphic concepts.

B. Clinical Description of the Syndrome

The episodic behavior dyscontrol disorder is reported to present characteristic clinical features, which one can classify into: a) episodic and b) interepisodic disturbances.

(1) Episodic Disturbances

The most striking characteristic of this disorder is the occurrence of paroxysmal behavioral disturbances, which develop suddenly, cease spontaneously, and exhibit a conspicuous tendency to recurrence. These maladaptive behavioral events generally occur spontaneously or more often, with minimal environmental provocation, and are out of character for the individual and out of context for the situation, and grossly out of proportion to the triggering events that elicited the reaction. Behavior associated with these episodes is perceived by the patient as ego dystonic, evoking guilt and remorse, and appearing to be beyond conscious volitional control or unconscious motivating processes. The more or less paroxysmal character of these episodes is reminiscent of an epileptic seizure. The patient often describes the episodes as "spells" or "attacks", primarily because they are delimited by a precipitous onset and outset, and are disruptive to his life-style as an ego-alien experience. The behavior during the episodes lacks adaptive value for the individual and shows impaired degrees of goal-directedness and coordination, and absence of significant anticipatory planning and premeditation. The symptoms occur more or less suddenly, within minutes or hours, and very often with an explosive character, and remit almost as quickly.

The most common behavioral disturbance during these episodes involves explosive outbursts of anger, and/or loss of control of aggressive impulses, resulting in violent and often destructive behavior. Aggression occurring during these episodes is primarily expressive rather than instrumental, and involves the display of intense affects of anger which may result in serious assault or destruction of property. This affective aggression is primarily directed towards "significant others," such as friends and relatives rather than strangers. In general, the expression of affective violence during these episodes is characterized by impulsivity and hair-trigger explosivity in the form of violent emotional outbursts. Following an episode, the patient expresses genuine regret and self-reproach at the consequences of his behavior, and acknowledges impaired capacity to control his aggressive impulses (41). The occurrences of impulsive violent acts during the episode may lead to the criminalization of these individuals. Violence in criminal behavior, however, is not necessarily an indication of the presence of episodic dyscontrol. In our experience, the majority of individuals suffering from episodic dyscontrol have a history of noncriminalized behavioral disturbances, and only a minority of them have had law-breaking encounters. The likely reason for the paucity of criminalized acts in these individuals seems to be associated with the observation that their aggression is generally expressed affectively within the tolerant atmosphere of the family situation, and that it rarely results in bodily harm, and when it does, it rarely leads to the completion of a judicial process resulting in conviction.

Nevertheless, although aggressive episodes of a violent nature represent a dramatic and striking feature of this disorder, it appears that this criterion may be absent in many cases, and when it is present, it is generally associated with other disturbances, both episodic and interepisodic. The new diagnostic category of "Intermittent Explosive Behavior" in the DSM III defines only those patients whose episodic dyscontrol is characterized by loss of control of aggressive impulses which results in serious assault or destruction of property. This diagnostic category is, therefore, restrictive and fails to include those patients who show episodic behavior disorder other than aggressive behavior dyscontrol. As a matter of fact, many of these patients show a broad range of other episodically occurring disturbances, including episodes of depression which is often associated with self-destructive behavior, sometimes in the form of "suicidal fits," episodes of emotional excitement, fits of running away during an emotional outburst, and impulsive acts, such as racing a car. Other symptoms which may be associated with the occurrence of these episodes and which appear to be suggestive of an epileptic-like character include: prodromal autonomic sensations and affective symptoms of irritability and mounting tension signaling an impending episode, subtle changes in the level of consciousness suggestive of impaired awareness during the episode and partial amnesia of the events surrounding the episode. These amnesic, confusional, or dissociative-like symptoms may be absent, and are not, therefore, considered essential for the diagnosis of this disorder. In addition to these episodic disturbances, some authors have included into the syndrome more sustained behavioral disturbances of a psychotic nature, both schizophreniform and affective.

(2) Interepisodic Disturbances

An important clinical feature of this syndrome is that there is no evidence of generalized impulsivity or aggressiveness between episodes, a feature which is thought to differentiate this disorder from the diagnosis of "explosive personality." Nevertheless, it is believed that patients suffering from this disorder show evidence of additional psychopathology between episodes, which remains largely unexplored. A significant number of these patients are found to have "soft" neurological signs, suggesting the presence of organic disturbance, such as memory disturbances (forgetfulness), hypersensitivity to sensory input (e.g., hyperacousis or photosensitivity), awkwardness and accident proneness. Hypochondriasis is a commonly reported symptom. There is very little known about the personality structure and organization of these patients. Monroe's

Episodic Dyscontrol Disorders

(41) extensive study on the psychodynamic aspects of these patients is obscured by inadequately defined criteria in the selection of these patients, and a broadening of his concept of "episodic behavior disorders" to an extent that the syndrome appears to lose in specificity.

In our experience with such patients, it appears that alcoholism and drug abuse may significantly be associated with the episodic dyscontrol syndrome, an observation that needs further substantiation. It is of interest that the reported neuropsychological and EEG disturbances in polydrug abusers, which have been attributed to the use of these drugs, may have pre-existed to a large extent, and may have been responsible for the occurrence of substance abuse (17).

Developmental pathology reported to be present in the history of these patients includes hyperactivity, aggressiveness, temper tantrums, and enuresis in childhood, and aggressive or delinquent behavior during adolescence, as well as a history of brain injury. The suggestion that minimal brain dysfunction and dyscontrol syndromes may share a common mechanism of brain dysfunction is most interesting and deserves careful evaluation. The observation that both syndromes are more common among males adds further plausibility to this notion. On the other hand, there is very little evidence to support an epileptic etiology in the MBD syndrome, a fact that conflicts with the prevailing assumptions of an epileptic mechanism for the dyscontrol syndrome.

In a recently published study on incarcerated aggressive criminals, Monroe, Balis, Lion, and associates (44) were able to define, on the basis of a self-rated dyscontrol scale and activated EEG theta waves, an episodic dyscontrol group which was designated as "epileptoid," and another group labelled as "inadequate psychopath." Both groups manifested evidence of CNS dysfunction revealed by an activated EEG (chloralose-induced theta abnormalities); however, the "epileptoid" group rated high on episodic dyscontrol, while the "inadequate psychopath" group was low on that scale. It was found that the "epileptoid" group could be identified by other measuring instruments as long as they consisted of data from the neurological examination, psychiatric history, current behavior, and psychometric tests. Among measures distinguishing the "epileptoid" group from the others, a neurological scale consisting of eleven items provided a score that differentiated this target group from all others. This neurological scale included a history of possible 1) birth trauma, 2) head injury, 3) formes frustes of epilepsy, and 4) CNS insult, such as infection, and excessive drug use. The neurological examination contributed to this score in terms of physical evidence of 1) congenital stigmata, 2) hyperacousis, 3) photophobia, 4) apraxia, and 5) asymmetries in motor strength. On the other hand, this group actually performed better than the other groups on 6) gross coordination, and 7) sensory discrimination, contrary to expectations. The "inadequate psychopath" group, (low dyscontrol behavior), in spite of the presence of the same EEG evidence of brain dysfunction, showed lack of neurological signs and symptoms (except for the EEG theta), and minimal psychometric evidence for organicity. This group, was identified, however, by the psychiatric history, particularly by such factors as poor adaptation to stress, impaired judgment, emotional unresponsiveness, hypersensitivity, fluctuation of feelings, lack of responsibility, grandiosity, aimlessness, alcohol abuse, brooding, agitation, and severity of symptoms. This group appeared to be the most severely ill and socially deviant one. In spite of the EEG evidence of CNS dysfunction, this group showed no history of brain "insult" during early childhood. It was reasoned that the brain dysfunction in this group reflected a "maturational lag," whereas, the brain dysfunction in the "epileptoid" group reflected an "epileptoid" mechanism. It is very likely that what differentiates these two groups is not the presence of the dyscontrol syndrome but the history of brain injury. We suspect that the so-called "epileptoid" group is a mixed one consisting of subjects having CNS dysfunction due to brain injury in early childhood, as well as subjects whose CNS dysfunction is due to some type of other etiology, referred to by the authors as "maturational lag." Subjects having the latter brain dysfunction may or may not show an episodic dyscontrol disorder, depending on factors that await clarification. We would like to point out here that, the episodic dyscontrol syndrome does not appear to represent a single homogeneous nosological syndrome, and therefore, it is premature to elevate it to a specific diagnostic entity. Furthermore, its etiology remains obscure, in spite of claims to the contrary. It is clear that it consists of several subgroups which differ both clinically and etiologically, as well as with regard to response to treatment. The great majority of these patients are not known to suffer from clinical epilepsy—at least according to criteria acceptable to epileptologists. The EEG of these patients is generally normal or shows nonspecific abnormalities, particularly in the form of slow activity (theta-delta). Some of these patients may show specific EEG abnormalities, such as hypersynchrony, isolated spikes and sharp waves, or localized slow waves. The nonspecific abnormalities have variously been interpreted as being suggestive of brain organicity, paroxysmal disorder, CNS dysfunction, CNS instability, or reflecting a maturational lag. Only a small minority of these patients show involvement of the temporal lobe regions, an observation that fails to support the correlation of the syndrome with temporal lobe epilepsy or temporal lobe syndrome. Some investigators have tried to improve the diagnostic efficacy of the EEG by the use of specialized activating procedures, including Metrazol, photic stimulation, intravenous Brevital, and alpha chloralose activation.

Monroe and Balis (44) have used alpha chloralose as an effective activating EEG procedure in the diagnosis of episodic dyscontrol disorders. Alpha chloralose appears to elicit two types of EEG abnormalities in these patients: a) specific or categorical EEG abnormalities, such as spikes, hypersynchrony, or focal slow waves, suggestive of epilepsy and/or organic brain damage; these abnormalities are most frequently seen in patients known to suffer from epilepsy, however, the majority of patients with episodic dyscontrol fail to show specific abnormalities: b) non-specific EEG abnormalities, characterized by slow activity, which occurs: 1) either as low to moderate amplitude diffuse or scattered theta, or 2) as paroxysmal bursts of high amplitude rhythmic slow wave activity, primarily within the delta range, which is bilaterally synchronous and symmetrical and with a frontal preponderance. This non-specific slow-wave response to chloralose activation occurs with equally high prevalence (75-80%) in both epilepsy and episodic dyscontrol; the same activation pattern also occurs in approximately 20% of the general population, thus indicating that this abnormality itself is not a sufficient etiological factor in the development of episodic dyscontrol disorders. It has been suggested that the nonspecific slow-wave response to alpha chloralose activation may be indicative of an underlying CNS instability which is assumed to play an important role in the mechanism underlying the episodic disorders. However, the description of the presumed brain dysfunction as representing "CNS instability" leaves one with many unanswered questions: How one defines CNS instability? What is the neurophysiological mechanism of this so-called instability? Is CNS instability related to epileptic predisposition or epilepsy, and if so, in what way? Or, is CNS instability a general dysfunctional state of the brain that cuts across many clinical syndromes? And finally, what is the mechanism of the slow-wave response to chloralose, and how is this related to the mechanism of CNS instability? These are

Psychotropic Drug Research

basic questions that need to be answered in order to begin to understand the neurophysiological mechanisms which underlie the dysfunctional state of episodic dyscontrol, to recognize their possible interconnection with other clinical syndromes, and thus find effective ways to treat them.

III. EFFECT OF DRUGS IN EPISODIC DYSCONTROL DISORDERS

There is very little known about the treatment of episodic dyscontrol disorders. Most of the available literature deals with the therapeutic control of violence in patients suspected or diagnosed to have temporal lobe epilepsy or limbic system disorders. A number of neurosurgical procedures (temporal lobotomy, amygdalectomy, cingulotomy) have been used with variable results in the treatment of episodic aggression, especially when it is associated with demonstrably specific etiology (tumors, vascular abnormalities, harmatomata, mesial incisural sclerosis). However, patients with specific etiological diagnoses should not be included in the episodic behavior dyscontrol disorder. This disorder, as defined in the DSM III under the diagnosis of "Intermittent Explosive Disorder," belongs to Axis II which includes diagnostic categories of nonspecific etiology. The concept of "Intermittent Explosive Disorder" is closest to the target syndrome under consideration, although it is too narrowly defined by restricting the disorder to an exclusively aggressive impulse dyscontrol. Since most of the literature does not differentiate this nonspecific diagnosis from those with a specific etiology (e.g., brain tumor, epilepsy), it is not possible, at present, to determine which of the recommended methods are effective in the treatment of this disorder. The following review will be limited to the effect of various drugs in the treatment of the episodic dyscontrol disorders of nonspecific etiology. It is clear that, since most of the investigators are heavily biased by the presumed "epileptoid" character of the disorder, the major focus of interest in the literature has been on the effects of various anti-epileptic drugs. Other pharmacological agents that have been given a trial on an empirical basis, include benzodiazepines, phenothiazines, tricyclic antidepressants, lithium, stimulants, and others.

Most available studies are methodologically unacceptable, either because of inadequately defined patient groups, or because of lack of double-blind procedures, insufficient population samples, and other deficiencies in methodological design. Most of these studies are uncontrolled or anecdotal case reports attempting to assess the effect of drugs on a great variety of patient populations on the basis of some ill-defined criterion that is assumed to reflect an epileptic mechanism, such as episodicity, aggressiveness, impulsivity, "soft" neurological signs, or nonspecific EEG abnormalities. These patients represent the full range of psychiatric nosology, including schizophrenia, both acute and chronic, affective disorders, personality disorders, psychoneuroses, organic brain syndromes, childhood hyperactivity (MBD), and so forth.

A. Anti-epileptic Drugs

Diphenylhydantoin (Dilantin®), alone, or in combination with other anti-epileptic drugs (i.e., primidone), benzodiazepines, or neuroleptics, is the most frequently recommended drug. Studies dealing with the use of diphenylhydantoin alone refer primarily to the effect of the drug on undifferentiated behavioral disorders (30), behavioral concomitants of epilepsy (43), severely psychotic aggressive patients (41), hostility scores in chronic hospitalized schizophrenics (57), and other syndromes which have obviously very little in common, and only a tenuous relationship with the episodic behavior dyscontrol disorder as defined. Monroe (41) contends that diphenylhydantoin would be effective only in episodic disorders, and then only in those with an epileptoid mechanism, and recommends it as the first drug regimen to be tried when such a mechanism is clearly established. He bases these assertions on inferences from studies in related disorders and from his own uncontrolled studies and case reports. Phenylhydantoin has been used in combination with chlordiazepoxide and primidone for uncontrolled psychotic patients (43) with some positive results; in combination with neuroleptics in chronic schizophrenic females (48) with a reported reduction in irritable aggressive behavior; in combination with phenobarbital in the treatment of neurotic patients with a reported lessening of irrascibility and compulsiveness (65); and in combination with methylphenidate in delinquent boys with no significant differences between drug and placebo groups (10). Again, none of these reports involve controlled studies of the target syndrome. Carbamazepine (Tegretol®) and primidone (Mysoline®), alone or in combination with other drugs, have also been recommended in the treatment of episodic dyscontrol disorders (41, 42, 44, 55), on the basis of inferences drawn from the effects of these drugs on the behavioral disturbances of epileptic patients. Carbamazepine is an anti-epileptic agent reported to exert a psychotropic effect in epilepsy as well as in other conditions. A number of studies report favorable results with regard to the use of carbamazepine in the treatment of epileptic children with behavior disorders (including aggressiveness and impulsivity) (49), as well as in non-epileptic children with behavior disorders (18, 27, 52), and non-epileptic adults (16). Groh (18) reports beneficial effects with carbamazepine in a group of non-epileptic children who were described as labile in mood, irritable, dysphoric, reacting violently to the slightest provocation and showing unpredictable reactions and abnormal EEG recordings. These patients showed what he describes as the "erethistic-hyperkinetic" syndrome, implying a concept of masked or latent epilepsy. This group closely resembles the episodic behavior dyscontrol of adult patients. Similarly, Kuhn-Gebhart (27) reports favorable results with the use of carbamazepine in a group of non-epileptic children who showed a variety of symptoms including hyperkinesia, aggressiveness, antisocial acts, enuresis, autonomic nervous disturbances, as well as abnormal EEGs characterized by considerable irregularity with a pronounced tendency to theta and delta activity, and with hypersynchronous phases of slow activity in response to hyperventilation. He comments: "Broadly speaking, the more abnormal the EEG findings, the greater the likelihood that anti-epileptic treatment will prove successful." Again, Kuhn-Gebhart's group of children show significant similarities with the adult manifestations of episodic behavior dyscontrol. In a discussion of the psychotropic effects of carbamazepine in non-epileptic adults, Kuhn (26) finds carbamazepine effective not only in controlling the unrestrained emotional outbursts and mood changes in epileptics, but also in patients to whom the term "epileptoid" is sometimes applied. He suggests that the prospects of a favorable response are best in those cases which show a pattern of symptoms suggestive of some underlying cerebro-organic cause or in which the EEG tracings deviate from normal. Tunks (62) identifies the dyscontrol syndrome as a limbic system dysfunction which requires a drug regimen that raises seizural threshold; she finds a favorable response to carbamazepine in patients with a diffuse and nonspecifically abnormal EEG and who show no clinical evidence of epilepsy. Several authors have pointed out that the chemical structure of carbamazepine is akin to that of the iminodibenzyl compounds and that this group might be a promising source in the development of drugs for the treatment of the dyscontrol syndrome (26, 62).

There have been very few studies with regard to the use of primidone in the treatment of episodic dyscontrol. An earlier study by Monroe (43) reported that primidone alone or in combination with other drugs controlled impulsive aggressive behavior in uncontrolled psychotic patients. In a recently published study by Monroe, Balis, and associates (44) in a group of incarcerated aggressive criminals, primidone was found to be ineffective in controlling symptoms of dyscontrol behavior as measured by infraction ratings. The failure was attributed to the insensitivity of the criterion and to the short observation period (6 weeks).

It is reasonable to conclude that a number of patients with episodic dyscontrol syndrome may improve on a regimen of anti-epileptic drugs, especially those showing evidence of serious EEG abnormalities suggestive of a presumptive diagnosis of epilepsy and brain organicity. There is definite need for well-designed controlled studies that would pay attention to the methodological problems concerning the delineation of several etiologically different subgroups within this syndromatic category, and which may respond differentially to various regimens of drugs. Therapeutic trials with established, as well as newly introduced anti-epileptic drugs, alone or in combination, are needed, with an emphasis on differential responsiveness.

B. Benzodiazepines

Benzodiazepines (chlordiazepoxide, diazepam, oxazepam, clonazepam), given alone or in combination with anticonvulsant drugs, have also been reported to be effective in the treatment of dyscontrol patients (23, 31, 41, 53). Chlordiazepoxide (Librium®), alone or in combination with anticonvulsants, was reported to normalize the abnormal EEG of long term schizophrenic patients, with greater improvement of behavior being observed in those patients whose EEG had been normalized (41, 42). This drug was also reported to be particularly effective in aggressive impulsive women (53). Beneficial effects in episodic dyscontrol patients have also been reported with the use of diazepam (Valium®). It has been suggested (44) that oxazepam (Serax®) may be a more specific "hostility tranquilizer" than other benzodiazepines, in view of the reported observation that this drug does not increase anger, hostility, and aggressiveness as other benzodiazepines do. Unfortunately, there are no adequately done studies that demonstrate the postulated effectiveness of the various benzodiazepines in the treatment of episodic dyscontrol. The need for such studies is stressed in view of the recent evidence that most of the ben-

Psychotropic Drug Research

zodiazepine actions are probably compatible with a theory focused on aminobutyric acid (GABA)-mediated potentiation of pre-and postsynaptic inhibition (60). GABA is a major inhibitory neurotransmitter in the brain, especially in the cerebral cortex, that may be regulating descending cortical inhibitory tone on subcortical structures, including limbic system. At brain stem, GABA appears to mediate a presynaptic inhibition, a mechanism that could modulate and reduce the amount of incoming sensory information (60). Besides GABA, neurotransmitters displaying prominent interactions with benzodiazepines include glycine, norepinephrine and serotonin. Diazepam preferentially antagonizes seizures associated with a reduction in the biosynthesis of GABA (60).

C. Lithium

Several preliminary studies have shown that lithium can have an inhibitory effect on impulsive aggressive behavior, and therefore, one might expect that it could be useful in the treatment of at least some forms of episodic dyscontrol syndrome (3, 11, 33, 58, 59, 63, 64). Most of these studies report to the effectiveness of lithium in preventing aggressive-violent outbursts in heterogeneous groups of prisoners diagnosed as having personality disorder, epilepsy, brain injury, or psychosis. Sheard (58, 59) has found in single-blind and double-blind studies involving prisoners that lithium exerts an inhibiting effect on chronic human aggressive behavior. In Tupin's (64) nonblind study, subjects were described as an extremely manipulative, hostile, and aggressive group who were extroverted, highly impulsive, and action-oriented, and with an MMPI profile showing peaking on psychopathic deviate, and manic scales, and extremely high scores on hostility. In a report by Atschuler (3) involving nine patients who had various diagnoses but shared-in-common symptoms of impulsivity and aggression, Lithium® seemed to affect the target symptoms of impulsivity and aggressiveness, regardless of diagnosis. In view of this array of diagnoses, common underlying features have been suggested, including: a) undiagnosed atypical affective disorder; b) family history of affective illness; and c) affective elements apparent in the illness (11, 33, 59). Tupin (63) suggests, on the basis of available evidence, that there is a common underlying neurophysiological disturbance which is behaviorally manifested in the following ways: "1) extreme stimulus sensitivity—a "hairtrigger," 2) the inability to reflect on the meaning or intent of the stimulus, i.e., the lack of reflective, intro-

208

spective review to assess accidental or purposeful attack, and 3) maximal response—little capacity to modulate the expression of anger." The same behavioral triad has also been reported to characterize patients with episodic dyscontrol (41). It appears that, although lithium may have some general effect on impulsive aggressiveness, patients with affective aggressiveness suggestive of an atypical manifestation of manic-depressive illness may be the most responsive group. This is typically exemplified by a case report (11) of a 30-year-old man with a five-year history of impulsive, violent, and assaultive episodes during which he felt "like exploding," and who had no evidence of epilepsy or organicity; further evaluation revealed a history of mood swings that led to the diagnosis of bipolar manic-depressive illness. Lithium treatment resulted in marked improvement of the episodic disturbances. It was thought that the episodes of impulsive assault may suggest a "switch mechanism" similar to that reported to characterize some bipolar patients who change rapidly from depression to mania (8, 54). One may further postulate that the reported aggravation of dyscontrol behavior of patients treated with tricyclics may not be due to an activation of an "epileptoid" mechanism, as suggested by Monroe (41), but to the activation of the "switch mechanism" that leads to an atypical "manic shift" (8).

Aggressive children with various diagnoses, as well as children with hyperactivity, have been noted to improve with lithium treatment. These preliminary studies await confirmation.

We are as much impressed by the affective character (intense affects and emotions) of many patients with episodic behavior dyscontrol, as we are by their impulsive aggressiveness. It is clear that the effects of lithium in the episodic dyscontrol syndrome demand careful consideration, with particular attention on the differentiation of etiologically disparate subgroups, and the eventual elimination of those patients with a specific etiological diagnosis, such as bipolar affective disorder. Through this process of differential elimination of etiologically known subtypes, we may finally be able to abolish completely this provisional syndromatic category. One should also note that lithium appears to affect diverse systems in the brain, and that, therefore, it may prove useful in clinical conditions which differ etiologically. Recent research suggests that lithium may have a multiplicity of actions, i.e., it decreases release and increases re-uptake of norepinephrine; it alters the release, uptake, and synthesis of serotonin; it alters transport of glucose, amino acids, and other cations across cell mem-

Psychotropic Drug Research

branes; it competes with calcium and magnesium ions and therefore, may alter calcium-dependent neuronal functions and their
modulation by magnesium; finally, it alters adenyl cyclase activity
and cyclic AMP levels, which are believed to be components of
neurotransmitter receptors.

D. Tricyclic and Stimulant Drugs

Very little is known about the effect of tricyclic antidepressants in
these disorders. There are only anecdotal or isolated case reports
which present conflicting findings (2, 19, 32, 41, 45). Tricyclics are
thought by some to exacerbate symptoms or precipitate seizures in
these patients (41), thus suggesting that they intensify an epileptoid mechanism. Although this may be true for patients whose
episodic dyscontrol represents ictal phenomena, it may also be
likely that the exacerbation of the episodic disturbances of some of
these patients may involve a "switch mechanism" in an atypical
bipolar affective disorder, in which affective aggressiveness may be
thought of as equivalent to a "manic shift" (8). It is of interest that
tricyclic antidepressants, as well as CNS stimulants (d-amphetamine, methylphenidate, or pemoline) have been reported by others
to produce beneficial effects in patients whose episodic dyscontrol is
associated with a history of minimal brain dysfunction (hyperactivity) in childhood (2, 19, 32, 45). Thus a report by Morrison
(45) on a group of adult subjects with "explosive personality" and a
history of hyperactivity in childhood indicates that these patients
showed a favorable response to tricyclics. The proposed notion of
"adult brain dysfunction (ABD)," as a sequela of childhood MBD,
which is thought to exist alone or with a variety of other psychiatric
symptoms, has led some clinicians to try in addition to imipramine,
various stimulants with satisfactory results (2, 19, 32). It is thought
that these drugs may lead to improvement in impulse control and
in the disordered attention fundamental to MBD. Of the earlier
authors, Hill (22) followed for more than four years eight violent
psychopathic patients treated with amphetamines. His patients
had a history of hyperactivity in childhood, a family history of
epilepsy, late enuresis, very deep sleep, and diffusely abnormal
EEGs. Hill found that the personalities which respond are those
showing an aggressive, bad-tempered, and generally hostile tendency. However, he found that "The most satisfactory patients are
those predominantly aggresive characters capable of a warm interpersonal relationship, but continually wrecking such relationships."

210

Episodic Dyscontrol Disorders

The reported high incidence of drug abuse in patients with episodic dyscontrol and MBD, may suggest a pattern of self-medication as a means of controlling dysphoric feelings and impulsivity. One may conclude that, in spite of the reported successful use of tricyclic and stimulant drugs in a number of recent studies involving isolated cases, it is not possible, at present, to assess the usefulness of these drugs in patients with episodic dyscontrol.

E. Other Drugs of Potential Usefulness

(1) Neuroleptics (i.e., phenothiazines)

These drugs have been used in episodic dyscontrol patients with variable results. Some authors report that many of these patients tend to deteriorate when placed on neuroleptics, a phenomenon that has been attributed to the effect of these drugs in augmenting EEG abnormalities and lowering convulsive threshold (41). Others report that in adults and children with behavioral disorders accompanied by epileptic-looking EEGs, anticonvulsants are effective, but otherwise phenothiazines are to be preferred.

(2) Propranolol

This beta-adrenergic blocking agent was found by Elliot (13) to be useful for controlling aggressive behavior following brain damage. This report is of particular interest in the light of recently published preliminary studies indicating that this drug might be effective in the treatment of some forms of acute schizophrenia, as well as in post-partum psychosis, manic psychosis, and psychosis associated with porphyria (4). According to Atsmon and Blum (4), the psychotic symptomatology which responded to propranolol consisted of anxiety, excitement, disturbances in thought processes, disturbances in affect, and hallucinations; this symptom complex, called the "hyper-beta syndrome," was worsened by the use of phenoxybenzamine. Conversely, it was found that symptoms consisting of tension, withdrawal, outbursts of rage and psychomotor activity with low threshold to external stimuli (referred to as the "hyper-alpha syndrome"), were improved by the alpha blockers phenoxybenzamine or phentolamine. In some patients the "hyper-alpha syndrome" was unmasked when full blockage of the "hyper-beta syndrome" was reached. The authors suggest that the "hyper-alpha syndrome," which appears to largely resemble the dyscontrol

211

Psychotropic Drug Research

syndrome, could probably be delineated and treated with alpha-receptor blocking drugs.

(3) Progesterone (Provera®) and Testosterone Antagonists

These drugs may prove to have some usefulness in the treatment of some forms of aggressive dyscontrol, in the light of recent research suggesting that some components of aggressive and sexual behavior in man may be organized and regulated by a steroid-sensitive neural pathway. There is evidence indicating that sexual aggressive behavior of subhuman primates and lower mammals may be testosterone-dependent when testosterone is experimentally manipulated. However, the relationship between testosterone and human aggressive behavior remains unclear, in view of conflicting reports in the literature, suggesting positive (12, 47) as well as negative correlations (25, 39, 40). In a review of this subject, Rose (56) concludes that "Those *few* men who are at the extreme of the population in terms of early history of more aggressive and violent crimes, chronic aggressive behavior before as well as in prison, or the most violent and brutal rapists, tended to have higher testosterone values when compared with other prisoners or normal controls. It is possible that increased testosterone levels might play some role, clearly not simple cause and effect, but perhaps in concert with other factors in leading to these extremes of aggressive behavior." It would be of interest to study the adjunct use of testosterone antagonists as a means of manipulating the testosterone-dependent propensity to aggressive behavior.

(4) Opioid Peptides (enkephalins and endorphins) and Their Antagonists (i.e., naloxone)

Much excitement has been generated by the recent discovery of stereospecific opiate binding sites ("receptors") in the brain, coupled with the isolation, purification, and subsequent synthesis of the several naturally occurring opioid peptides, the enkephalins and endorphins. There is already significant evidence regarding the distribution and subcellular localization of these peptides, as well as the projections of neurons containing peptides to various regions of the brain. It has been postulated (7) that the potent behavioral changes induced by β-endorphin in rats might make these peptides potential etiological factors in some mental illness, and that opiate antagonists might offer some therapeutic benefit if this view were valid. Some recent electrophysiological and EEG findings regarding the effects of opiate peptides appear to be particularly relevant to conceptual and experimental approaches to the understanding and treatment of episodic dyscontrol disorders. Single unit studies (46, 69) in the rat show that enkephalin and endorphins exert an inhibitory effect on cerebral cortex, brainstem, caudate nucleus, and thalamus; in contrast, hippocampal pyramidal cells, and spinal cord Renshaw cells are mainly excited by these peptides. It has been further found that both inhibitory and excitatory effects could be antagonized by naloxone (46). More recent studies have focused on the unexpected excitation seen in the hippocampus (16). Opiate peptides as well as opiate alkaloids have been reported to alter spontaneous EEG patterns in both animals and man. Endorphins are powerful epileptogenic agents, and can produce these EEG effects at molar doses far less than comparable doses of the opiate alkaloids. What appears to be of particular interest is the reported observation in rats that although EEG seizures are precipitated by β-endorphin, behavioral convulsions are not seen following either acute or chronic administration (21). Most importantly, the seizural activity seems to be primarily restricted to the limbic structures, and appears not to extend into motor systems. Repeated injections of beta-endorphin results in an attenuation of the epileptic response suggesting the development of tolerance (or perhaps inhibition). At higher doses of beta-endorphin the EEG shows cortical synchrony and slow wave activity as well as interictal spikes while the animal shows marked behavioral rigidity. This synchronous activity can be desynchronized by minimally arousing stimuli. The entire EEG response can be reversed or blocked by the administration of the specific opiate antagonist naloxone, before or subsequent to the emergence of the discharges. The limbic localization of these paroxysmal discharges without spreading, together with the cortical hypersynchrony and slow wave activity, seem to provide a model of the so-called "limbic system disorder" that is presumed to underlie the episodic dyscontrol syndrome. The use of naloxone in the treatment of this disorder may potentially prove to have beneficial effects for some patients.

IV. SOME PRELIMINARY RESULTS IN DEFINING SUBTYPES OF EPISODIC DYSCONTROL DISORDERS

It is clear that these disorders do not appear to be clinically or etiologically homogeneous, but rather represent a conglomerate of component syndromes having diverse etiology and pathogenesis,

Psychotropic Drug Research

and presumably differential responsiveness to treatment. In order to be able to study the effect of drugs and other therapies in these patients, it is necessary that we first delineate characteristic clinical subtypes that may have different etiology. With this consideration, we are presenting the following preliminary data from our laboratory that demonstrate the differentiation of several subgroups based on electroencephalographic findings.

A. Patient Samples and Methodology

Our population consists of patients referred to us by practicing psychiatrists for assessment of minimal brain dysfunction through the use of chloralose-activated EEGs and the evaluation of relevant clinical data. The majority of these patients present episodic dyscontrol disorders and are suspected of having an epileptoid disturbance or some other form of brain dysfunction. Known epileptics or patients with typical epileptic seizures are rarely referred to our laboratory, since the diagnosis of epilepsy in such patients is established by standard methods elsewhere. We have found these patients ideal for the study of episodic dyscontrol disorders, because they represent a highly selected group screened by physicians who are quite knowledgeable of this syndrome. The referring physician fills a form that provides us with a range of data, including a brief description of the presenting problem with particular emphasis on episodic dyscontrol acts, history of brain injury, neurological examination and laboratory findings, clinical diagnosis, and current medications. In addition, the patient fills a self-reporting neuropsychological inventory, which we have specially constructed as a means of obtaining data with regard to the following areas: a) episodic psychopathology; b) non-episodic psychopathology, which is further divided into neuropsychophysiological disturbances, personality assessment, and psychopathology; c) family and developmental pathology, with a focus on family history of epilepsy and episodic dyscontrol, history of brain injury, and developmental psychopathology limited to data supporting a presumptive diagnosis of minimal brain dysfunction during childhood and adolescence. This inventory consists of over 550 questions, organized in sets of five or multiples of five items and which constitute scales purporting to measure the presence or absence of a certain clinical variable. Each question has face validity from a clinician's point of view, since they represent questions asked by physicians to elicit pertinent pathology, and in which a positive answer could be considered contributory to forming a presumptive clinical judgment. The scales concerning the episodic psychopathology are constructed on a four-point basis, and the remaining on a true-false basis.

The EEG procedure includes: a) a standard baseline record utilizing ten montages with the international system of electrode placement (22 electrodes), and consisting of both bipolar and monopolar to the ipsilateral ear recordings, with a total duration lasting 30-45 minutes; b) a chloralose-activated record which is obtained 45 minutes after the per os administration of alpha chloralose (3 mg per pound of body weight), with a total duration lasting another 30-45 minutes. The analysis of EEG data is based on the narrative report of the electroencephalographer. Baseline and activation abnormalities were classified as two distinct types following the example of Ajmone-Marsan. The first type is designated as "specific" (or categorical) abnormalities and include focal slow wave activity, transient spikes or sharp waves (either focal or random), spike-slow wave activity, and hypersynchrony (focal or generalized). The second type is designated as "nonspecific" and is further differentiated into two subtypes: a) low to moderate voltage 5-7 cps nonrhythmic activity (theta), which appears scattered or diffuse; and b) bursts of high voltage 1-3 cps rhythmic activity (delta), which is bilateral synchronous and with a frontal preponderance.

Up to now we have collected data on a total of 120 cases. In this report we are presenting data on a total of 32 cases collected last year and subjected to a preliminary analysis. The original sample contained 34 subjects, of whom one was eliminated because of a high score on the lie scale of the self-reporting questionnaire, and a second one was eliminated because he was a single case of 6 and 14 cps positive spike discharges to be placed under a separate category. Patients were divided into four groups, on the basis of EEG abnormalities as follows: 1) *Normal EEG Group:* Subjects show a normal EEG in both baseline and chloralose-activated recordings; 2) *Categorical Group:* Subjects show "specific" EEG abnormalities revealed in the baseline and/or the chloralose-activated recordings; 3) *Theta Group:* Subjects show chloralose-induced (activated recordings) nonspecific EEG abnormality consisting of low to moderate voltage 5-7 cps nonrhythmic activity (theta), which appears to be scattered or diffuse; 4) *Delta Group:* Subjects show chloralose-induced (activated recordings) nonspecific EEG abnormality consisting of bursts of high voltage 1-3 cps rhythmic activity, which is bilateral, synchronous, and with a frontal predominance. Each of these groups contains eight subjects (total of 32 cases). In addition, the three groups with EEG abnormalities (Categorical, Theta, and Delta) were grouped into one category (Group with Abnormal EEGs).

B. Results

Table I summarizes various demographic data, clinical diagnoses, and EEG abnormalities, for each of the designated EEG groups. The majority of the subjects are males in the Abnormal EEG groups (75 to 100%), as compared to the normal EEG group (63%). Most subjects are young adults with a mean age for each group ranging from 26 years (Normal EEG and Delta) and 30 years (Categorical, Theta). There is very little difference in the age range of each group (15 to 43 years). Of the 32 subjects, only one is black. There are no marked group differences with regard to marital status, except for the Delta group (13% married as compared to 25% in the Categorical and 38% in the Theta and Normal EEG groups). There are no significant group differences in the level of education, although the Theta and Delta groups show somewhat higher levels.

With regard to clinical diagnoses, 67% of the subjects in the Abnormal EEG groups, and 75% of the Normal EEG group were reported to show episodic dyscontrol acts of an aggressive-violent nature. The remaining subjects were referred for screening out suspected CNS dysfunction. A psychotic diagnosis was made in 38% of the Categorical group (two schizophrenics, one affective psychosis) and 12% in the Delta group (one paranoid psychosis). No psychotic diagnoses were made in the Theta and Normal EEG groups; 50% of the subjects in the latter groups were diagnosed as suffering from psychoneuroses. The Delta group had a variety of diagnoses with a predominance of personality disorders (38%). The Theta group had a predominance of psychoneuroses (50%) and personality disorders (38%). The Categorical group had a variety of diagnoses, with a predominance of psychoses (38%). The Normal EEG group consisted only of psychoneuroses and personality disorders. Twenty percent of the subjects in the Abnormal EEG groups were given the diagnosis of organic brain syndrome.

With regard to EEG abnormalities, of the 32 subjects 15% had an abnormal baseline record while 75% had EEG abnormalities in either baseline or chloralose-activated records. This finding confirms once more the usefulness of alpha-chloralose activation as a means of eliciting evidence of brain dysfunction. The Categorical group showed the following specific EEG abnormalities; 63% of the

TABLE I
Four group classifications based on EEG abnormalities.

Demographic Data	Group Differentiation by EEG (reported in % except for age)				
	Normal EEG N=8	Abnorm. EEG N=24	Categorical* N=8	Theta* N=8	Delta* N=8
Sex: Males	63	88	100	88	75
Mean Age	26	29	30	30	26
Age Range	15 - 39	19 - 43	18 - 43	19 - 36	15 - 39
Mar. Status: 1) Married	38	25	25	38	13
2) Other (Sing. Sep. Divorc.)	62	75	75	42	87
Education: 1) Jr. & Sr. High School	75	67	75	63	63
2) College & Grad. School	25	33	25	37	37
Clinical Diagnoses					
Episodic Dyscontrol (Violent)	75	67	75	63	66
Psychoses (Schiz., Paran., Affective)	0	17	38	0	12
Psychoneuroses	50	29	12	50	25
Personality Disorders	50	21	25	38	38
Organic Brain Syndrome	0	20	25	12	25
EEG Abnormalities					

TABLE I Continued

Baseline Abnormalities:	0	21	63	0	0
Lt. temporal focus hypersynchr.	0	8	25	0	0
Rt. temporal focus slow waves	0	8	25	0	0
High voltage rhythmic delta	0	5	13	0	0
Chloralose-Activated Abnormalities	0	100	100	100	100
High voltage rhythmic delta	0	58	75	0	100
Low-moderate voltage theta	0	33	0	100	0
Bilateral hypersynchrony	0	13	38	0	0
Focal temporal hypersynchrony	0	4	13	0	0
Focal temporal rhythmic delta	0	8	25	0	0

*

1) Categorical Group: 100% specific EEG abnormalities revealed in the baseline and chloralose-activated records.

2) Theta Group: 100% nonspecific EEG abnormalities, induced by chloralose activation, and consisting of low to moderate voltage 5-7 cps nonrhythmic activity, which appears scattered or diffuse.

3) Delta Group: 100% nonspecific EEG abnormalities, induced by chloralose activation, and consisting of bursts of high voltage 1-3 cps rhythmic activity, which is bilateral, synchronous and with frontal preponderance.

subjects had baseline abnormalities, consisting of left temporal focus hypersynchrony (25%), right temporal focus slow waves (25%), and high voltage rhythmic delta (13%); additional abnormalities elicited by chloralose activation included: high voltage rhythmic delta (75%), bilateral hypersynchrony (38%), focal temporal hypersynchrony (13%), and focal temporal rhythmic delta (25%).

Table II summarizes data from the self-reporting inventory describing episodic psychopathology in each of the four groups. These preliminary data (presented as percentages of subjects scoring to the criterion) show in a striking manner that patients with a normal EEG differ significantly in many respects from those showing abnormal EEG recordings. With regard to episodic dyscontrol involving aggressive-violent behavior, the abnormal EEG subjects score much higher, especially with regard to "anger-aggressiveness, experienced only" (92% vs 37%); the latter includes items such as, feeling like smashing things, urge to do something harmful, feeling angry enough to kill someone, feeling cross without any reason, and worrying about losing control of urge to hurt someone. However, there are differences among the three groups with the EEG abnormalities, with the Categorical group showing fewer episodes of unprovoked or minimally provoked violent acts. It is clear that subjects in the Delta and especially the Theta groups are more violent and potentially dangerous.

An important finding in Table II is that subjects with EEG abnormalities experience, at a high incidence, a number of other episodic dyscontrol disturbances, including spontaneous episodes of fear-panic, elation, depression, unprovoked suicidal attempts, racing cars recklessly, sexual excitement, and voracious eating. However, there are significant differences among the three groups with abnormal EEGs: The Delta group shows no suicidal attempts, and is rather low in episodes of elation, reckless driving, and voracious eating. The Theta group shows again the highest scores in all items, while the Categorical group is low in episodes of fear-panic and suicidal attempts.

Another significant finding is that all three abnormal EEG groups show a high incidence of dysmesic episodic disturbances, characterized by impaired consciousness during the episode and subsequent amnesia of the events surrounding it. These episodes include fugue-like states in which the subject behaves in strange ways or automatically without awareness, (especially the Categorical and Theta groups), violent dyscontrol episodes associated with amnesia

TABLE II
Episodic psychopathology.

Episodic Dyscontrol (violence)	Group Differentiation by EEG (% of subjects scoring to the criterion)				
	Normal EEG N=8	Abnorm. EEG N=24	Categorical N=8	Theta N=8	Delta N=8
Violent episodic dyscontrol—total	37	96	87	100	100
Episodes of violence, unprovoked	25	42	25	62	50
Episodes of violence, triggered	37	50	37	62	50
Anger-aggressiveness, experienced only	37	92	87	100	87
Other Episodic Dyscontrol Disturb.					
Episodes of fear-panic, spontaneous	0	38	12	50	50
Episodes of elation, spontaneous	0	29	50	25	12
Episodes of depression, spontaneous	12	54	50	50	62
Suicidal attempts, unprovoked	12	17	12	37	0
Racing car recklessly	12	46	50	62	25
Episodes of sexual excitement	12	42	37	50	37
Episodes of voracious eating	0	33	37	37	25
Dysmnesic Episodic Disturbances					
Fugue-like episodes	12	54	62	62	37
Violent dysmnesic episodes	12	42	62	37	12

Momentary absences	0	42	37	25	62
Grand mal seizures	0	4	12	0	0
Dysmnesic disturbances, Total	12	71	75	62	75
Episodic Perceptual Disturbances					
Illusory visual	25	79	75	75	87
Illusory auditory	0	42	50	37	50
Depersonalization-derealization	12	42	25	37	62
Deja vu	50	42	25	50	50
Hallucinatory-like experiences	12	63	62	37	87
Other Episodic Disturbances					
Sudden sense of extreme loneliness	12	79	87	75	62
Sudden sense of extreme happiness	0	36	62	12	37
As if everything occurred in rhythm	0	17	37	0	12
Paroxysmal autonomic episodes	50	75	75	87	62
"Organic-like" Episodes					
Drug-induced confusional episodes	0	54	75	62	25
Miscellaneous "organic" episodes	25	63	62	87	37

(Categorical group, and to a lesser extent Theta group), and momentary absences (very prominent in the Delta group). It appears that subjects in the Delta group experience primarily petit mal-like periods of absence (62%), while the subjects in the Theta and Categorical groups experience primarily fugue-like episodes (62%). In addition, the Categorical group shows violent dysmnesic episodes (62%), and grand mal seizures (12%).

Furthermore, subjects in the three groups with EEG abnormalities show a high incidence of episodic perceptual disturbances. Visual illusory experiences (79%) are particularly prominent in the Delta group (87%), and are described as: surroundings acquire strange qualities, things seem pulsating, walls or ceilings appear to be closing in, things look unreally remote or too close, things look enormously enlarged, things seem receding or approaching, things look unreally minute, and feelings of dream-like detachment. Auditory illusory experiences (42%) are described as: sounds or voices acquire bizarre quality, become distant or whispering, unbearably loud or close, or becoming hollow. Depersonalization-derealization experiences (42%) are particularly prominent in the Delta group (62%) and are described as episodes of "feeling detached from surroundings" and "detached from body, unreal body, floating." Hallucinatory-like experiences (63%) are particularly prominent in the Delta (87%) and the Categorical groups (62%) and are described as: hearing unreal sounds (bells, drumming, etc.), hearing voices, experiencing vivid visions, and smelling foul odors. The Delta group appears to be the most prone to experiencing episodic perceptual disturbances.

Another episodic disturbance reported at a very high incidence by the subjects in all three groups with EEG abnormalities is episodes of a sudden sense of extreme loneliness (79%); subjects in the Categorical group also reported a high incidence (62%) of episodes of sudden sense of extreme happiness, as well as feelings "as if everything occurred in rhythm" (37%).

Another striking finding is that the Categorical and Theta groups differ significantly from the Delta group, and much more so from the Normal EEG group, with regard to episodes labelled as "organic-like." Specifically, the Categorical and Theta groups show high incidence of drug- or alcohol-induced confusional episodes (75% and 62%), described as pathological intoxication, as well as febrile deliria (37% and 25%). Furthermore, these two groups also show a very high incidence of what we have designated as "miscellaneous organic episodes" (62% and 87%), described as episodes of slurred speech (75% and 62%), episodes of dropping things (62% and 62%), episodes of loss of balance (50% and 100%), and episodes of dizziness (50% and 62%). The Delta group shows only 25% of the subjects reporting drug- or alcohol-induced confusional episodes, and 37% of miscellaneous "organic" episodes. These data provide evidence indicating that the "organic" etiology characterizes primarily the Theta and Categorical groups, while the Delta group stands out as a distinguishable dysfunctional group of presumably different etiology.

Table III presents data regarding the non-episodic psychopathology (interepisodic) disturbances. When the three abnormal EEG groups are combined together they show higher rates in most items as compared to the Normal EEG group. Specifically, these subjects score higher on hypochondriasis, autonomic instability, inattention-distractibility, orientation disturbances, forgetfulness, incoordination, impaired arousal-alertness, hyperacousis, photophobia, hypersexuality, and sleep walking. The Normal EEG group shows high scores on insomnia and hyposexuality. There are also significant differences among the three groups with EEG abnormalities, which further contribute to their differentiation as discrete syndromes. The Delta group shows in general lower scores than the other two, and therefore, it appears less pathological; relatively higher scores occur in hypochondriasis, forgetfulness, hyperacousis, photophobia, and hypersexuality. The Theta group scores again as the most pathological in most variables, including hypochondriasis, autonomic instability, inattention-distractibility, forgetfulness, impaired arousal-alertness, uncoordination (poor at sports, accident prone), hyperacousis, hypersexuality, recurrent dreams, sleep walking and sleep disturbances. The Categorical group stands in general, between the Delta and Theta groups, with regard to degree of pathology; it shows an unusually high incidence of sleep walking (37%). The Categorical and Theta groups differ from the Delta group, in that they show higher incidence of inattention-distractibility, forgetfulness, uncoordination, sleep walking, recurrent dreams, sleep deficit, and sleep excess. Once more, these two groups appear to be more "organic" than the Delta group.

With regard to personality, the Normal EEG group shows a large number of subjects who score high in obsessive-compulsive traits (50%), passivity (50%), and emotional excitability-intense affects (50%). The three abnormal EEG groups, when combined together, contain subjects who score high (46%-75%) on almost all personality scales, with the exception of passivity. This perversive psy-

TABLE III

Nonepisodic psychopathology.

Neuropsychophysiological Disturb.	Group Differentiation by EEG (% of subjects scoring to the criterion)				
	Normal EEG N=8	Abnorm. EEG N=24	Categorical N=8	Theta N=8	Delta N=8
Hypochondriasis	12	50	37	62	50
Autonomic instability	12	42	25	62	37
Attention-concentration disturbances	37	50	62	50	37
Orientation disturbances	12	33	37	25	37
Forgetfulness	25	83	87	100	62
Incoordination, Total	0	38	50	62	0
Poor at sports	0	38	50	62	0
Accident prone	0	33	50	50	0
Impaired arousal-alertness	25	54	37	87	37
Difficulty in thinking clearly	12	50	25	87	37
Mind feels "foggy"	25	38	12	50	50
Hyperacousis	25	50	50	50	50
Photophobia	25	37	37	37	37
Hypersexuality	12	54	50	62	50
Hyposexuality	50	33	37	37	25
Sleep walking	0	21	37	25	0
Recurrent dreams	37	42	37	75	12
Sleep deficit (insomnia)	87	58	75	62	37
Sleep excess	37	50	62	50	37

Personality Psychopathology-Traits

Obsessive-compulsive traits	50	67	75	87	37
Paranoid traits	25	58	37	78	62
Schizoid-introverted traits	25	46	37	75	25
Passivity traits	50	17	12	37	0
Social unconcern-self-centeredness	25	50	50	37	62
Labile object relationships	12	50	37	50	62
Extraversion traits	37	63	75	50	62
Hypomanic traits	12	46	50	50	37
Emotional excitability-intense affects	50	75	75	75	75
Histrionic, attention seeking	12	63	75	62	50
Emotional lability	12	50	62	62	25
Impulsivity	12	67	75	50	75
Ego-dystonic impulsive acts	25	58	37	87	50

Personality Psychopathology-Symptoms

Obsessive-compulsive symptoms	12	50	37	62	50
Paranoid symptoms	25	50	50	62	37
Schizophrenic-like symptoms	12	58	50	75	50
Phobic symptoms	25	46	25	62	50
Depressive symptoms	37	67	62	87	50
Anxiety symptoms	37	63	75	75	50
Alcoholism	37	50	37	75	37
Drug abuse	25	54	50	37	75

chopathology involves both pre-psychotic and polyneurotic personality traits, reminiscent of borderline personality organization. On the other hand, there are significant individual differences in each of the three groups with EEG abnormalities, with the Theta showing the highest score in most scales, and with the Delta appearing as the least pathological. The Categorical and Theta groups contain subjects who score very high in obsessive-compulsive traits, hypomanic traits, and emotional lability. The Theta group shows the most polymorphous psychopathology, and is further distinguished from the other groups by high scores on schizoid-introverted traits and strong ego-dystonic attitude towards their impulsive acts (87%). Impulsivity is highest in the Categorical and Delta groups (75%), and somewhat lower in the Theta group (50%). The Categorical group contains subjects who score low on paranoid and schizoid traits (37%), passivity (12%), labile object relationships, and ego-dystonic impulsive acts. On the other hand, the Delta group contains subjects who score high in paranoid traits, social unconcern-self-centeredness, labile object relationships, extraversion, emotional excitability-intense affects, histrionic and attention-seeking behavior, and impulsivity; conversely, these subjects score low in obsessive-compulsive and schizoid traits, passivity (0%), hypomanic traits, and emotional lability. This group seems to present a profile that closely resembles that of a sociopathic individual.

Symptomatic psychopathology is elevated in all scales when the three groups with abnormal EEG are combined together, and as compared with the Normal EEG group. Their profile is again one of polysymptomatic neurosis, characterized by, obsessive-compulsive symptoms, phobias, anxiety and depressive symptoms, which are coupled with pre-psychotic personality structures, including, paranoid schizoid and hypomanic personalities. In addition, these subjects report high incidence in alcoholism (50%) and drug abuse (54%), and as it was mentioned earlier, high incidence in episodic dyscontrol (poor impulse control), intense affects, especially with regard to anger-hostility, dissociative reactions, and especially fugue states and amnesia accompanied by disturbances of consciousness, intense sense of extreme loneliness, and hypochondriasis. This psychopathology also represents the salient features of the Borderline Personality (Unstable Personality Disorder). The following significant differences are noted among the three groups with abnormal EEGs. The Delta group shows very high scores in drug abuse (75%), while the Theta group shows very high scores in alcoholism (75%). The Theta group emerges once more as the most pathological one, with highest scores in depression (87%), schizophrenic-like symptoms (75%), and anxiety symptoms (75%).

Table IV shows data from the self-reporting questionnaire describing family history of epilepsy and episodic behavior disorders, history of brain injury, and developmental pathology with a focus of a childhood history of MBD. With regard to a family history of epilepsy, only the Categorical and Theta groups scored high (37%). Interestingly, the Theta group reported a history of epilepsy only among siblings and offsprings, which seems to suggest prenatal and perinatal factors as one possible etiology. With regard to the family history of episodic behavioral disturbances, we find again that the Categorical and Theta groups show the highest incidence (twice that of Delta and Normal EEG groups). These findings strongly suggest that the Categorical and Theta groups are associated with a genetically or familial predisposition to epilepsy.

The findings regarding the history of brain injury are again striking with the Theta and Categorical groups showing an incidence of 87% and 100%, correspondingly, for serious head trauma. The Delta group shows a 25% incidence and the Normal EEG group 36%. The latter finding indicates that one third of the subjects of the Normal EEG group have a serious history of head trauma associated with loss of consciousness. Therefore, it is possible that this is not a purely functional group, in spite of the fact that it does not show EEG abnormalities. In addition to head injury, the Categorical group is also characterized by a high incidence of "prenatal insult" (repeated abortions, serious complications during pregnancy, major illness during pregnancy, difficult labor, and Caesarian section), perinatal and postnatal "insult" ("very sick baby" when born, prematurity, incubator care, head injuries during labor), serious childhood infections (repeated middle ear infections, severe case of measles, rheumatic fever, febrile convulsions and chorea), and toxic-metabolic conditions (carbon monoxide poisoning, dangerous exposure to poisonous chemicals, and serious hypertension). The Theta group shows, in addition to head trauma, a high incidence of serious childhood infections and toxic-metabolic conditions. These findings further confirm the observation that the Categorical and Theta groups involve a significant amount of "organicity," while the Delta group does not. Furthermore, there is suggestion that the subjects in the Categorical group may have had an early exposure to head injury, before or during birth or early childhood. The same can be said about the Theta group, although to a lesser extent. Finally, the findings regarding a history of MBD

TABLE IV
Family history-developmental pathology.

	Group Differentiation by EEG (% of subjects scoring to the criterion)				
Family History of Epilepsy	Normal EEG N=8	Abnorm. EEG N=24	Categorical N=8	Theta N=8	Delta N=8
Family history of epilepsy, total	0	29	37	37	12
Paternal side	0	8	25	0	0
Maternal side	0	13	25	0	12
Siblings & offsprings	0	17	12	37	0
Family H/O Episodic Disturbances	22	44	50	56	25
Blackouts	25	38	62	25	25
Confusional episodes	0	33	37	62	0
Episodes of loss of self-control	25	58	62	75	37
Episodes of violent behavior	37	46	37	62	37
H/O episodic disturbance, total	22	44	50	56	25
History of Brain Injury					
Prenatal "insult"	25	29	50	25	12
Perinatal and postnatal "insult"	25	21	37	12	12
Serious childhood infections	12	63	87	62	37
CNS infections	0	8	12	0	12
Serious head trauma	36	71	87	100	25
Toxic-metabolic conditions	12	46	62	50	25

History of MBD and Hyperactivity

H/O MBD, total	62	78	37	59	12
MBD suspect-infancy ("irritable baby")	12	12	37	21	0
MBD suspect-preschool ("difficult toddler")	75	62	75	71	12
MBD suspect ("hyperactive child")	62	62	75	67	37
Unable to sit still	62	50	62	58	37
Constantly fiddling with things	62	50	75	63	25
Behavior problem-aggressiveness	87	87	50	75	12
Prone to temper tantrums	50	62	50	54	25
Easily provoked to fighting	62	75	37	58	25
Passive aggressiveness	50	87	37	58	12
Disobedience	37	50	12	33	12
Sassiness	50	62	12	42	23
Behavior problem-antisocial	62	25	12	33	37
Fire-setting	62	25	12	33	37
Animal cruelty	75	25	12	38	37
Incoordination-awkwardness	37	37	50	42	37
Poor at sports	12	25	50	29	12
Accident prone	0	25	25	17	12
Inattention-distractibility	50	37	50	46	25
Learning difficulties	75	75	75	75	50
Difficulty in learning arithmetic	12	50	75	46	12
Enuresis	50	25	50	42	12
Adolescent behavior problem—delinquency	100	87	50	79	25
Expelled or suspended from school	25	37	50	38	25
Involvement of juvenile court	50	12	25	33	0
Incarceration in institutions	25	0	0	8	0

Psychotropic Drug Research

and hyperactivity in childhood seem to support the reports of other investigators about a high incidence of this syndrome in patients with episodic dyscontrol. When the three abnormal EEG groups are combined together, the difference between them and the Normal EEG group in the total MBD scale is 59% vs 12%. This means that about 60% of subjects with episodic dyscontrol disorder and an abnormal EEG have a retrospective history of childhood MBD. If one examines the MBD subscales, he would note the same significant differences, with subjects in the abnormal EEG group reporting a high incidence on "irritable baby" 21% (colicky, crying constantly, difficult to soothe, problem with sleep); "difficult toddler" 71% (strong willed and demanding, constantly "into everything," "did not listen," speech problem); hyperactive child 67% (unable to sit still, constantly touching and fiddling with things, unable to stop moving all the time, unable to stop talking all the time); behavior problem-aggressiveness, 75% (temper tantrums, easily provoked to fighting, constantly punished-discipline problem); passive aggressiveness, 58% (disobedient, stubborn, very sassy); inattention-distractibility, 46% (unable to concentrate, easily distracted, unable to follow directions); learning difficulties, 75%; enuresis, 42%; and adolescent behavior problem-delinquency, 79%. In all of the above subscales, these patients showed significantly higher scores than those in the normal EEG group.

Once more, we observe that there are significant differences among the three groups with EEG abnormalities. In the total MBD scale, the Theta group shows the highest incidence (78%), and the Categorical the lowest (37%). The incidence for the Delta group is 62%. The Delta group, compared to the other groups, shows significantly higher scores on the following MBD subscales: fire-setting (62%), animal cruelty (75%), and adolescent behavior problem-delinquency (100%), especially with regard to involvement in the juvenile courts (50%) and incarcerations in institutions (25%). In this regard, the Delta group appears again to stand out by its high incidence of serious behavior problems in childhood, and serious delinquency in adolescence, presenting early indication of antisocial behavior. The Categorical and Theta groups differ from the Delta group in that they show low incidence of antisocial behavior during childhood and adolescence, and high incidence of uncoordination, 50% (especially poor at sports, and accident prone), and learning difficulties with a characteristic problem in learning arithmetic.

V. CONCLUSION AND DISCUSSION

A review of the concept of Episodic Dyscontrol Disorder reveals

230

that this is not a clinically or etiologically homogenous syndrome, and that, therefore, it is not possible, at present, to make any firm statement about the action of drugs in the treatment of this disorder. In order to be able to study the effect of drugs and other therapies in these patients, it is necessary that we first delineate distinguishable clinical subtypes that may have different etiology, and presumably differential responsiveness to treatment. In the light of this consideration, we presented some preliminary results from our laboratory, which clearly suggest that it is possible to classify patients with episodic dyscontrol in at least four clinically distinguishable groups, on the basis of using chloralose-activated EEG abnormalities as the initial criterion for grouping. More specifically, these data show that patients with a normal EEG differ significantly from those showing EEG abnormalities elicited by a chloralose-activation procedure. Furthermore, patients with EEG abnormalities differ clinically according to whether their activated EEG shows specific (categorical) abnormalities, nonspecific-nonrhythmic theta, or nonspecific-rhythmic delta activity.

Group 1 (normal EEG) seems to contain subjects whose episodic dyscontrol behavior is primarily psychologically determined, and who are usually diagnosed as suffering from personality disorders or psychoneuroses. In order to obtain a more homogenous sample, one should exclude subjects with a history of serious brain injury, even in the absence of EEG abnormalities or any other evidence of "organicity."

The "psychogenic" group does not seem to represent a distinguishable diagnostic category. It contains a spectrum of clinical diagnoses within the range of psychoneuroses and personality disorders and clearly excludes psychoses and organic brain syndromes. The episodic dyscontrol behavior is symptomatic to the underlying psychological disturbance and is clearly not associated with clinical or EEG evidence of brain dysfunction. There is no family history of epilepsy and no history of brain injury. They have very few psychophysiological complaints, except for complaints of forgetfulness, lightheadedness, insomnia, and hyposexuality. They have no history of hyperactivity in childhood, except for learning difficulties. In personality, they tend to show a clustering of traits around an obsessive-compulsive organization (especially with regard to need for anticipatory control, orderliness and structuring of their environment), appear to be emotionally excitable, with strong emotions, and show a proclivity to passivity (giving up easily when thwarted, suggestible).

Psychotropic Drug Research

Group 2 (categorical EEG abnormalities), group 3 (nonspecific nonrhythmic theta), and group 4 (nonspecific-rhythmic delta) have in common presumptive evidence of CNS dysfunction, which, however, differs etiologically in each group. Clinically, they have the following features in common. With regard to episodic psychopathology, they show a range of episodically occurring disturbances, including: a) violent dyscontrol episodes, often unprovoked or minimally provoked; b) other episodic disturbances, such as spontaneous episodes of depression; c) episodic perceptual disturbances, primarily of an illusory nature and similar to those reported by temporal lobe epileptics as aural experiences; d) dysmnesic episodes, suggestive of dissociative (fugue) reactions during which there is impaired level of consciousness; and e) paroxysmal autonomic episodes. With regard to non-episodic psychophysiological disturbances, these subjects show: a) hypersexuality (strong sexual desires which they find hard to control); b) forgetfulness; and c) hyperacousis. Regarding nonepisodic personality psychopathology, they tend to show: a) obsessional characteristics (with regard to anticipatory control, orderliness and structuring of the environment); b) extraversion; c) schizoid experiences, possibly related to the bizzare perceptual distortions which occur episodically; d) depressive symptoms; e) intense affects associated with emotional excitability, and especially intense anger which presents an explosive threat; f) a hysterical proclivity to dramatization, acting out and attention-seeking behavior; and g) impulsivity, the consequences of which are ego dystonic. Finally, they also share in common a history of childhood psychopathology which is strongly suggestive of MBD, including descriptions of "difficult toddler," "hyperactivity," behavior problems associated with aggressiveness, learning difficulties, and adolescent behavior problems.

Groups 2 and 3 (Categorical and Theta) present some significant similarities which are not shared by Group 4 (Delta), and which clearly distinguish them from the latter. Specifically, they share: a) a history of brain injury (especially with regard to serious head trauma, serious childhood infections, and toxic-metabolic conditions); b) a history of disturbances commonly interpreted as "soft" neurological signs, and including inattention-distractibility, uncoordination (poor at sports, accident prone), drug- and alcohol-induced confusional episodes (pathological intoxication), and episodes associated with slurred speech, dropping things, loss of balance and dizziness; c) a family history of epilepsy and episodic dyscontrol disorders, with a suggestion that Group 3 reports a history of epilepsy only in siblings and offsprings; d) sleep disturbances (insomnia and sleep excess); e) emotional lability; f) hypomanic traits with mood swings; g) paranoid trends; h) dogmatism and authoritarianism; i) serious anxiety symptoms; and k) sleep walking. It is clear that these two groups have an organic etiology, and an epileptic predisposition which, however, is prominent only in Group 2 that shows categorical paroxysmal EEG discharges. It is likely that Group 3 is primarily organic and Group 2 is organic-epileptic. Most importantly, the two groups differ significantly with regard to the seriousness and amount of psychopathology, which is much greater in Group 3. It is primarily the additional pathology found in Group 3 that provides differentiating significance.

Group 2 shows, nevertheless, the following positive pathology that distinguishes it from Group 3: Subjects report in excess a history of prenatal and postnatal CNS "insult" and more serious head injuries; they are described as slow learners and underachievers in school, much more awkward and poor at sports, and with more serious attention problems; they also report a history of enuresis; episodic disturbances are more often associated with impairment of consciousness and amnesia, and have in excess illusory and hallucinatory-like experiences, depersonalization, and episodes of elation. In personality, they appear more impulsive, self-centered and egotistical, and more prone to hypomanic swings. In general, they closely resemble the personality of temporal lobe epileptics.

Group 3 represents the most pathological group. In addition to the pathology that it shares with the other two groups, it is characterized by the following positive features: Episodic psychopathology includes an excess in unprovoked violent episodes, episodes of fear panic and sexual excitement, much more intense angry feelings, and more frequent amnesic episodes of violence. Nonepisodic psychophysiological disturbances include hypochondriasis, autonomic instability, impaired arousal-alertness (difficulty in thinking clearly), and vestibular hypersensitivity (lightheadedness and tendency to lose balance). Developmental history shows a higher incidence of MBD (75%) in childhood with prominence of aggressiveness (temper tantrums, fighting and destructive behavior), as well as passive-aggressiveness. In personality, they show a much more serious and perverse mixture of psychopathology, with a prominence in paranoid and schizoid traits, and a much stronger ego-dystonicity in reaction to impulsive behavior. The general clinical profile is suggestive of an organic involvement of the temporolimbic system (temporal lobe syndrome).

Psychotropic Drug Research

Group 4 (Delta) is uniquely different from Groups 2 and 3 in regard to the nature of the underlying CNS dysfunction. Subjects clearly lack evidence of any organic deficit in terms of a history of brain injury, "soft" neurological signs, or EEG abnormalities with standard procedures. The distinguishing criterion for brain dysfunction becomes manifest by the chloralose-activation procedure, and consists of bursts of high voltage rhythmic delta, which is bilateral and symmetrical and shows a frontal preponderance. This aspecific abnormality is clearly centrencephalic in origin and has a paroxysmal character. One may say that this group is analogous to idiopathic epilepsy, without necessarily being epileptic. This dysfunction is thought to reflect a "CNS instability," perhaps secondary to a "maturational lag." It is assumed to exist from birth, and may be constitutionally and perhaps genetically determined. It may be thought to be analogous to the "epileptic predisposition" and yet different. We have labelled this dysfunctional CNS state "dysleptic predisposition" in order to emphasize its distinct and yet epileptoid nature. It is assumed to represent a proclivity, vulnerability, or high risk factor, the presence of which may predispose an individual, during the developmental years, to a certain psychopathology, namely, childhood MBD, adolescent delinquency, and borderline personality (unstable personality disorder) or episodic dyscontrol disorder in the adult. The postulated "dysleptic predisposition" is not viewed as a causative factor in the development of the above mentioned syndromes, and may exist in an individual without any evidence of psychopathology. It connotes a specific neurophysiological concept that characterizes certain aspects of unstable equilibria in CNS homeostasis. It is postulated that the "steady state" of modulation of the neuronal activity which is maintained by various intrinsic processes of excitation and inhibition, is presumed to represent a dynamic integrative state whose vicissitudes greatly depend on the capacity of the system to maintain its stability. We further conceptualize this "steady state" as a continuum expressing "shifts" in the stability of the system; increased tendency to deviations in the direction of greater instability within the system defines a CNS state of vulnerability that predisposes to the development of certain disturbances of an oscillatory or episodic nature and which are accompanied by a deficit in the integrative processes of the brain. The underlying dysfunctional state of the "dysleptic predisposition" is unknown. It reflects a labile organization which is prone to episodic disruptions, clinically manifested as a condition of "stable instability." It is assumed that

234

Episodic Dyscontrol Disorders

CNS states associated with a "stable instability" also include the "epileptic predisposition," as well as structural damage to the brain manifested by the so-called "soft" neurological signs. What is a common feature in all these conditions is an unstable "steady state" which predisposes to a proclivity to oscillatory or episodic disturbances associated with a temporary failure of the integrative processes. Freides (15) has proposed the general concept of "diaphoria" to denote all conditions of unstable "steady state" characterized by "variability and inconsistency in patterning and control." One may further assume that during "shifts" towards the direction of greater instability, the dysfunctional CNS state that characterizes the "diaphoric" conditions may become associated with a compensatory reactive inhibition in other areas of the brain, and that these reactive inhibitory processes may account for a great deal of the psychopathology observed during these episodic "shifts." In the case of epileptic seizures, this reactive compensatory inhibition is manifested as "postictal" phenomena. With regard to the dysleptic predisposition, alpha-chloralose exerts a destabilizing (excitatory) influence on an already unstable equilibrium, and this destabilizing effect is manifested in the EEG by the characteristic delta response, which most likely represents an outcome of compensatory inhibitory processes, rather than paroxysmal discharges. One possible explanation may rest on the assumption that the initial effect of chloralose is to facilitate already unstable excitatory axodendritic synapses (probably through thalamic-induced recruiting potentials), whose active depolarization produces a shift towards greater instability followed by inhibitory axosomatic postsynaptic potentials in the deeper cortical layers, in the form of bursts of slow waves that reflect the compensatory inhibitory process.

Group 4, as revealed by the characteristic chloralose-induced EEG activation, differs from the other two groups in several other respects. With regard to the episodic psychopathology, these subjects are less prone to suicidal episodes, dysmnesic violent episodes, fugue states, and drug-induced confusional episodes. On the other hand, they more often tend to show momentary lapses of consciousness, depersonalization-derealization experiences, and hallucinatory-like phenomena. These subjects also show a high incidence of drug abuse (75%), and hypochondriasis. In personality, they appear to be less pathological than Group 3. Their developmental history reveals serious antisocial behavior during childhood (fire setting, animal cruelty) and adolescence (delinquency of serious nature).

Psychotropic Drug Research

These preliminary data, although inconclusive because of the limited number of cases, strongly support the reported association of childhood MBD with the adult episodic dyscontrol. They further provide suggestive support to the notion that many of the subjects may be characterized by a borderline personality organization, thus pointing up to a triadic syndrome associated with an underlying brain dysfunction, which can be classified into "dysleptic" (or idiopathic), "organic," and "organic-epileptic."

Progress in the study of the drug effects in these disorders cannot be made without further delineation of the component syndromes. Such research should be directed towards well differential subtypes rather than target symptoms (e.g., aggression, episodicity, etc.).

REFERENCES

1. Alpers, B.J.: Relation of the hypothalamus to disorders of personality. Report of a case. *Arch. Neurol. Psychiatry,* 38:291, 1937.

2. Arnold, L.E., Strobel, D., and Weisenberg, A.: Hyperactive adult: study of the "paradoxical" amphetamine response. *JAMA,* 222:693-694, 1972.

3. Atshuler, K.J., Abdullah, S., and Rainer, J.D.: Lithium and aggressive behavior in patients with early total deafness. *Dis. Nerv. Syst.,* 38:521, 1977.

4. Atsmon, A., and Blum, I.: The discovery. In E. Roberts, and P. Amacher (Eds.): *Propranolol and Schizophrenia,* Alan R. Liss, Inc., New York, 1978, pp. 5-38.

5. Bach-y-Rita, G., Lion, J., Climent, C.E., et al: Episodic dyscontrol: a study of 130 violent patients, *Am. J. Psychiatry,* 127:1473-1478, 1971.

6. Balis, G.U.: Behavior disorders associated with epilepsy. In G.U. Balis, et al. (Eds.): *Psychiatric Foundations of Medicine,* Vol 4, pp. 4-63., Butterworth Co., Boston, Mass, 1978.

7. Bloom, F.E., Segal, D., Ling, N., et al.: Endorphins: profound behavioral effects in rats suggest new etiological factors in mental illness. *Science,* 194:630-632, 1976.

8. Bunney, W.E., Jr.: The switch process in manic-depressive psychosis. *Ann. Intern. Med.,* 87:319-335, 1977.

9. Cantwell, D.P.: Psychiatric illness in the families of hyperactive children. *Arch. Gen. Psychiatry,* 27:414-417, 1972.

10. Conners, C.R. et al.: Treatment of young delinquent boys with diphenylhydantoin sodium and methylphenidate. *Arch. Gen. Psychiatry,* 24:156, 1971.

11. Cutler, N., and Heiser, J.F.: Retrospective diagnosis of hypomania following successful treatment of episodic violence with lithium: A case report. *Am. J. Psychiatry,* 135:753-754, 1978.

12. Ehrenkrantz, J., Bliss, E., and Sheard, M.H.: Plasma testosterone:

correlation with aggressive behavior and social dominance in man.*Psychosom. Med.,* 36:469-475, 1974.

13. Elliott, F.A.: Propranolol for the control of belligerent behavior following acute brain damage. *Ann. Neurol.,* 1:489, 1977.

14. Falconer, M.A.: Place of surgery for temporal lobe epilepsy during childhood. *Br. Med. J.,* 2:631, 1972.

15. Freides, D.: A new diagnostic scheme for disorders of behavior, emotions, and learning based on organism environment interaction. Part I and II. *Schizo. Bull.* 2:218, 1976.

16. French, E.D., Siggins, G.R., et al.: Iontophoresis of opiate alkaloids and endorphins accelerates hippocampal unit firing by a non-cholinergic mechanism; correlation with EEG seizures. *Neuroscience Abstr.* 3: 291, 1977.

17. Grant, I., and Judd, L.L.: Neuropsychological and EEG disturbances in polygraph users. *Am. J. Psychiatry,* 133:1039-1042, 1976.

18. Groh, C.: The psychotropic effect of Tegretol in non-epileptic children, with particular reference to the drug's interaction. In W. Biermeyer (Ed.): *Epileptic Seizure—Behavior—Pain,* University Park Press, Baltimore, 1976, pp. 259-263.

19. Gross, M.D., and Wilson, W.C.: *Minimal Brain Dysfunction.* Brunner/Mazel, New York, 1974.

20. Hartocollis, P.: The syndrome of minimal brain dysfunction in young adult patients. *Bull. Menninger Clin.,* 32:102-114, 1968.

21. Henriksen, S.J., Bloom, F.E. et al.: Induction of limbic seizure by endorphins and opiate alkaloids: electrophysiological and behavioral correlates. *Neuroscience Abstr.,* 3:293, 1977.

22. Hill, D.: Amphetamine in psychopathic states. *Br. J. Addict.,* 44:50-54, 1944.

23. Kick, H., and Dreyer, R.: Clinical procedures with clonazepam under particular conditions of psychomotor epilepsy (abstract). *Acta Neurol. Scand.,* 49:54, 1973.

24. Killefer, F.A., and Stern, W.E.: Chronic effects of hypothalamic injury: Report of a case of near total hypothalamic destruction resulting from removal of a graniopharyngioma. *Arch. Neurol.,* 22:419, 1970.

25. Kreuz, L.E., and Rose, R.M.: Assessment of aggressive behavior and plasma testosterone in a young criminal population. *Psychosom. Med.,* 34:321-322, 1972.

26. Kuhn, R.: The psychotropic effect of carbamazepine in non-epileptic adults, with particular reference to the drug's possible mechanism of action. In W. Biermeyer (Ed.): *Epileptic Seizure—Behavior—Pain,* University Park Press, Baltimore, 1976, pp. 268-271.

27. Kuhn-Beghart, V.: Behavioral disorders in non-epileptic children and their treatment with carbamazepine. In W. Biermeyer (Ed.): *Epileptic Seizure—Behavior—Pain,* University Park Press, Baltimore, 1976, pp. 264-267.

28. Laufer, M.W., Denhoff, E.: Hyperkinetic behavior syndrome in chil-

dren. *J. Pediat.,* 50:463-473, 1967.
29. Livingston, K.E.: Limbic system dysfunction induced by "kindling": its significance for psychiatry. In W.H. Sweet, et al. (Eds.): *Neurological Treatment in Psychiatry, Pain and Epilepsy,* University Park Press, Baltimore, 1977, pp. 63-75.
30. Lohrenz, J., Levy, L., and Davis, J.F.: Schizophrenia or epilepsy? A problem of differential diagnosis. *Compr. Psychiatry,* 3:54, 1962.
31. Lorimer, F.M.: Violent behavior and the electroencephalogram. *Clin. Electr.,* 3:193, 1972.
32. Mann, H.B., and Greenspan, S.I.: The identification and treatment of adult brain dysfunction. *Am. J. Psychiatry,* 133:1013-1017, 1976.
33. Marini, J.L., Sheard, M.H.: Antiaggressive effect of lithium in man. *Acta Psychiatr. Scand.,* 55:269-286, 1977.
34. Mark, V.H., and Ervin,F.R. *Violence and the Brain,* Harper & Row, New York, 1970.
35. Mark, V.H., Sweet, W., and Ervin, F.R.: Deep temporal lobe stimulation and destructive lesions in episodically violent temporal lobe epileptics. In W.S. Fields, and W.D. Sweet (Eds.): *Neural Bases of Violence and Aggression,* Warren H. Green, St. Louis, 1975.
36. Mendelson, W., Johnson, N., and Stewart, M.A.: Hyperactive children as teenagers: a follow-up study. *J. Nerv. Ment. Dis.,* 153:273-279, 1971.
37. Menkes, M., Row, J., and Menkes, J.: A five-year follow-up study of the hyperactive child with minimal brain dysfunction. *Pediatrics,* 39:393-399, 1967.
38. Menninger, K.: *The Vital Balance.* Viking Press, New York, 1963.
39. Meyer-Bahlburg, H.F.L., et al.: Aggressiveness and testosterone measures in man. *Psychosom. Med.,* 36:269-274, 1974.
40. Monti, P.M., Brown, W.A., and Corriveau, D.P.: Testosterone and components of aggressive and sexual behavior in man. *Am. J. Psychiatry,* 134:692-694, 1977.
41. Monroe, R.R.: *Episodic Behavior Disorders,* Harvard University Press, Cambridge, Mass., 1970.
42. Monroe, R.R.: Anticonvulsants in the treatment of aggression. *J. Nerv. Ment. Dis.,* 160:119-126, 1975.
43. Monroe, R.R., and Wise, S.: Combined phenothiazine, chlordiazepoxide, and primidone therapy for uncontrolled psychotic patients. *Am. J. Psychiatry,* 122:694, 1965.
44. Monroe, R.R.: *Brain Dysfunction in Aggressive Criminals.* Lexington Books, Mass., 1978.
45. Morrison, J.R., and Minkoff, K.: Explosive personality as a sequel to the hyperactive-child syndrome. *Compr. Psychiatry,* 16:343, 1975.
46. Nicoll, R.A., Siggins, G.R., et al.: Neuronal actions of endorphins and enkephalin among brain regions: a comparative microiontophoretic study. *Proc. Natl. Acad. Sci. U.S.A.,* 74:2584-2588, 1977.
47. Persky, H., Smith, K.D., and Basu, G.K.: Relation of psychologic measures of aggression and hostility to testosterone production in man.

Episodic Dyscontrol Disorders

Psychosom. Med., 33:265-277, 1971.

48. Pinto, A., Simopoulos, A.M., Uhlenhuth, E.H., et al: Responses of chronic schizophrenic females to a combination of diphenylhydantoin and neuroleptics: a double-blind study. *Compr. Psychiatry,* 16:529, 1975.

49. Puente, R.M.: The use of carbamazepine in the treatment of behavioral disorders in children. In W. Biermeyer (Ed.): *Epileptic Seizures—Behavior—Pain.* University Park Press, Baltimore, 1976, pp. 243-247.

50. Quitkin, F., and Klein, D.F.: Two behavioral syndromes in young adults related to possible minimal brain dysfunction. *J. Psychiat. Res.,* 7:131-142, 1969.

51. Reeves, A.G., and Plum, F.: Hyperphagia, rage and dementia accompanying a ventromedial hypothalamic neoplasm. *Arch. Neurol.,* 20: 616, 1969.

52. Remschmidt, H.: The psychotropic effect of carbamazepine in nonepileptic patients, with particular reference to problems posed by clinical studies in children with behavioral disorders. In W. Biermeyer (Ed.): *Epileptic Seizures—Behavior—Pain,* University Park Press, Baltimore, 1976, pp. 253-258.

53. Rickels, K., and Downing, R.: Chlordiazepoxide and hostility in anxious outpatients. *Am. J. Psychiatry,* 131:442, 1974.

54. Rifkin, A., Levitan, S.J., et al.: Emotionally unstable character disorder—a follow-up study: 1. Description of patient and outcome. *Biol. Psychiatry,* 4:65-79, 1972.

55. Rodin, E.A., Rim, C.S., et al.: A comparison of the effectiveness of primidone versus carbamazepine in epileptic outpatients. *J. Nerv. Ment. Dis.,* 163:41, 1976.

56. Rose, R.M.: Neuroendocrine correlates of sexual and aggressive behavior in humans. In M.A. Lipton, A. DiMascio and K.F. Killam, (Eds.): *Psychopharmacology: A Generation of Progress,* Raven Press, New York, 1978.

57. Simopoulos, A.M., et al.: Diphenylhydantoin effectiveness in treatment of chronic schizophrenics. *Am. J. Psychiatry,* 30:106, 1974.

58. Sheard, M.H.: The effect of lithium in the treatment of aggression. *J. Nerv. Ment. Dis.,* 160:108-118, 1975.

59. Sheard, M.H., Marini, J.L., Bridges, C.L., et al.: The effect of lithium on impulsive aggressive behavior in man. *Am. J. Psychiatry,* 13:1409-1413, 1976.

60. Snyder, S., Enna, S.J., and Young, A.B.: Brain mechanisms associated with therapeutic actions of benzodiazepines: focus on neurotransmitters. *Am. J. Psychiatry,* 134:662-664, 1977.

61. Steward, M.A.: The hyperactive child syndrome. *Am. J. Orthopsychiat.,* 36:861-967, 1966.

62. Tunks, E.R., and Dermer, S.W.: Carbamazepine in the dyscontrol syndrome associated with limbic system dysfunction. *J. Nerv. Ment. Dis.,*

Psychotropic Drug Research

164:56, 1977.

63. Tupin, J.P.: Usefulness of lithium for aggressiveness (letter to the editor). *Am. J. Psychiatry,* 135:1118, 1978.

64. Tupin, J.P., Smith, D.B., Clanon, T.L., et al.: The long-term use of lithium in aggressive prisoners. *Compr. Psychiatry,* 14:311-317, 1973.

65. Uhlenhuth, E.H., et al.: Diphenylhydantoin and phenobarbital in the relief of psychoneurotic symptoms. *Psychopharmacology,* 27:67, 1972.

66. Walter, R.D.: Violence and aggression: The state of the art. In N. Burch and H.I. Atshuler (Eds.): *Behavior and Brain Electrical Activity,* Plenum Press, New York, 1975, pp. 541-548.

67. Wender, P.H.: *Minimal Brain Dysfunction in Children.* John Wiley & Sons, New York, 1971.

68. Wood, D.R., Reimherr, F.W., Wender, P.H., et al.: Diagnosis and treatment of minimal brain dysfunction in adults. *Arch. Gen. Psychiatry,* 33:1453-1460, 1976.

69. Zieglgansberger, W., and Fry, J.P.: Actions of opioids on single neurons. In A. Hertz (Ed.): *Developments in Opiate Research,* Marcel Dekker, New York, 1978, (in press).

8

The Use and Misuse of Anxiolytics in the Violent, Aggressive Individual

CALVIN R. BROWN, M.D.

I. INTRODUCTION

The need for control of behavior in the chronically aggressive personality of many criminals is obvious and acute. In 1974, nearly 10,000 ten milligram Valium® tablets per month were being given in an attempt to control anxiety and hostile behavior in inmates at the Utah State Prison, Draper, Utah. We found in our experience at the Prison, that the use of Valium® had resulted in an increased aggressiveness and occasional paradoxical rage reactions. Hall (4) and Lion (6), had found similar results in their studies but no controlled study could be found in the literature using prisoners as subjects.

A review of the literature, including the Physicians Desk Reference, and the inserts from Roche and Wyeth, revealed some interesting differences between the actions of Valium® and Serax®.

Valium® (diazepam) is a benzodiazepine derivative developed through original Roche research. Chemically, diazepam is 7-chloro-1, 3-dihydro-1-methyl-5-phenyl-2H-1, 4-benzodiazepin-2-one. It is a colorless crystalline compound, insoluble in water and has a molecular weight of 284.74. Its structural formula is as follows:

In animals, diazepam appears to act on parts of the limbic system, the thalamus, and hypothalamus, and induces calming effects. Diazepam, unlike chlorpromazine and reserpine, has no demonstrable peripheral autonomic blocking action, nor does it produce extrapyramidal side effects; however, animals treated with diazepam do have a transient ataxia at higher doses. Valium® is useful in the symptomatic relief of tension and anxiety states resulting from stressful circumstances or whenever somatic complaints are concomitants of emotional factors. It is useful in psychoneurotic states manifested by tension, anxiety, apprehension, fatigue, depressive symptoms, or agitation.

Valium® has several adverse reactions. These include, drowsiness, fatigue, and ataxia, and less frequently, confusion, depression, dysarthria, headache, hypoactivity, slurred speech, syncope, tremor, vertigo and minor gastrointestinal, genitourinary, cardiovascular, and dermatological complaints. In addition, some paradoxical reactions such as acute hyperexcited states, anxiety, hallucinations, increased muscular spasticity, insomnia, rage reactions, sleep disturbance and stimulation have been reported. These paradoxical rage reactions seem to be more prominent in hostile and aggressive individuals. Valium® has a half-life of 6 to 8 hours and metabolizes into several by-products. The end product is oxazepam.

Serax® (oxazepam) is the first of a chemically new series of compounds, the 3-hydroxybenzodiazepinones. A new therapeutic agent providing versatility and flexibility in control of common emotional disturbances, the product exerts prompt action in a wide variety of disorders associated with anxiety, tension, agitation and irritability, and anxiety associated with depression. In tolerance and toxicity studies on several animal species, the product reveals significantly greater safety factors than related compounds, (chlordiazepoxide and diazepam) and manifests a wide separation of effective doses and doses inducing side effects.

Serax® is 7-chloro-1,3-dihydro-3-hydroxy-5-phenyl-2H-1,4 benzodiazepin-2-one. A white crystalline powder with a molecular weight of 288.7, its structural formula is as follows:

Use and Misuse of Anxiolytics

Acute oral dose LD_{50} in mice is greater than 5000 mg/kg compared to 800 mg/kg for a related compound (chlordiazepoxide). This product has a wide margin of safety in subacute toxicity studies in dogs as compared to related compounds such as chlordiazepoxide.

Serax® is indicated for the management and control of anxiety, tension, agitation, irritability, and related symptoms. Such symptoms are commonly seen in patients with a diagnosis of psychoneurotic reaction, psychophysiological reaction, personality disorder, or in patients with underlying organic disease. Anxiety associated with depression is also responsive to Serax® therapy.

Serax® also has some adverse reactions. The necessity for discontinuation of therapy due to undesirable effects has been rare, however. Transient mild drowsiness is commonly seen in the first few days of therapy. If it persists the dosage should be reduced. In a few instances, dizziness, vertigo, headache, and rarely syncope have occurred either alone or together with drowsiness. Mild paradoxical reactions, i.e., excitement, stimulation of affect, have been reported in psychiatric patients; these reactions may be secondary to relief of anxiety and usually appear in the first two weeks of therapy.

Although the following side reactions have not as yet been reported with oxazepam, they have occurred with related compounds (chlordiazepoxide and diazepam); paradoxical excitation with severe rage reactions, hallucinations, menstrual irregularities, change in EEG pattern, blood dyscrasias including agranulocytosis, blurred vision, diplopia, incontinence, stupor, disorientation, fever, and euphoria. Since Serax® is the final metabolic breakdown product of the benzodiazepines it is assumed that its remarkable lack of serious side effects including paradoxical rage reactions is in part due to the lack of a mixture of metabolites in the blood stream during its metabolism, such as would be found in the metabolism of diazepam. Another possibility of course is the fact that Serax® has a shorter half-life and therefore the accumulative effects of dosage would not be so marked on the individual idiosyncrasies, but our observed rage reactions did not seem to be either dose or time related. Paradoxical rage reactions in the prison were defined as violent and unusual outbursts of temper or outright violence to himself or others. This included assault, attempted suicide, self-mutilation, and attempted murder. During the period in which large amounts of Valium® were being used in the prison there seemed to be an excessive number of attacks both verbal and physical, on guards, other prisoners, and self-mutilations such as cuttings,

243

burnings, sputum injections, and attempted suicides. Our initial use of Serax® as a substitute for Valium® seemed to diminish these paradoxical reactions. It was this fact that prompted this study.

Valium® dependency had become an increasing problem at the prison since its introduction, and unauthorized use of Valium® was also becoming a problem, as evidenced by the fact that increasing numbers of prisoners were faking illness, palming medications, requesting higher doses, and selling Valium® in the corridors for higher and higher prices.

Recent reports in the literature had indicated that Serax® (oxazepam), introduced in 1967, has most of the necessary beneficial effects of Valium®, Librium® and the other benzodiazepines without the incidence of paradoxical rage reactions or increased hostility, that are apparent in these drugs (1, 3). An extensive search of the literature revealed a paucity of information comparing the two drugs and almost no information on their use in prisons. The Index Medicus, from 1960 to 1977, the University of Utah Medical Library, and the MEDLINE Data base file, sponsored by the National Library of Medicine in Bethesda, Maryland, were all used to gather basic data. From these data it appeared that the expected rage reactions in non-prisoner populations was about five percent.

Salzman, et al. (8) reviewed current studies in which Serax® was compared with two other benzodiazepines, Valium® and Librium®. Salzman's findings indicated that paradoxical rage reactions and increased hostility were extremely rare with Serax®, with excellent calming effect and diminished symptoms of anxiety, depression, irritability, and insomnia. Only 3 patients out of 100 exhibited paradoxical excitability with no evidence of increased hostility. Valium® was not used in Salzman's study as a comparison.

Several other authors reported similar findings. Warner (9) and Bobon (2) studied 52 patients on Serax® with dosages up to 50 mg. per day without evidence of hostility or rage in either acute or chronic use. Madelina (7) recorded 41 patients on Serax with dosages up to 50 mg per day for up to four months with no evidence of drug irritability or paradoxical rage reactions. Zucker (11) described 400 patients on Serax® out of which three were involved in a fight and one reported strange sensations within two weeks after administration. Gardos, et al. (3) reported a comparative study using Librium® and Serax® along with a placebo, in a controlled double-blind study extending over a six-month period. In this study, Serax® showed a definite decrease in hostile behavior and little effect of placebo as measured by psychological, personality, and hostility tests. Important to this finding was the fact that both Serax® and Librium® exhibited a paradoxical increase in anxiety in certain individuals with minimal initial anxiety. Di Mascio and Barrett (1) reported relative antianxiety effects of several minor tranquilizers, including Valium®, Librium®, Tranxene®, and Serax® in double-blind placebo controlled trials. These studies suggested the conclusion that Librium® produced an unexpected increase in hostile feelings among the student volunteer research subjects, who were high in anxiety. No such increase in hostility was observed with Serax®. Kochansky, *et al.* (5) once again observed an increase in hostility effects associated with 30 mg of Librium®. Serax® in daily doses of 45 mg over a one-week period was associated with a decrease of hostility attacks. These effects were measured by special questionnaires relating to the psychological aspects of hostility and kindness in the personality testing of these individuals. In Kochansky's study, it appeared that Serax® was a superior hostility tranquilizer as compared to Librium®.

The literature on Valium®, on the other hand, gave a different impression. Lion *et al.* (16) reported two cases in the Journal of Diseases of the Nervous System in which Valium® and Tranxene® caused severe paradoxical rage reactions. These case history studies add evidence to the fact that the benzodiazepines should be used cautiously in persons with basically aggressive personality disorders. Westermeyer *et al.* (10) published a cohort study on sociopathy and drug use in a young in-patient psychiatric population. Their methods were well-controlled, double-blind, and corrected for demographic characteristics. In his study, heavy drug use is strongly correlated with problematic social behavior and impaired social resources. There was a correlation between early illicit drug use and criminal sociopathic behavior. While this study did not use Valium® or Serax® exclusively, the similarity of the effects of illicit drugs and benzodiazepines on the young criminal sociopath was of interest to our study.

Hall (4) reported in the American Journal of Psychiatry, on a new syndrome called "Abnormal Response to Diazepam" which more resembled depression than rage, in which a number of patients who exhibited spontaneous weeping, confusion, decreased memory, and a drive to suicide, when taking more than 40 mg daily of Valium®, were studied. This paradoxical reaction may have been the same as the prison rage reactions but in less violent individuals.

Psychotropic Drug Research

II. Methods

From these reports in the literature and the high incidence of paradoxical reactions at the Utah State Prison, it became quite clear to us that Valium® was of questionable value in aggressive populations such as prisoners. However, some type of therapy was necessary for anxious persons incarcerated in a hostile and dangerous environment. Many inmates have anxiety related to problems outside the prison as well.

In the search for a more appropriate drug than Valium®, a double-blind, randomized study was designed to determine the difference between Valium® and Serax® as tranquilizers for inmates. A prospective therapeutic trial was initiated, using 100 inmates selected at random from the male population at the Utah State Prison, medium and minimum security sections. Only those patients who a physician or psychiatrist decided were in genuine need of tranquilization, were given Valium® or Serax® and neither the physician nor the patient knew which drug was being administered until after the study was completed. The drugs were dispensed by the prison pharmacist and delivered by trained medical technicians. No inmate was included in the series if he had been on any form of tranquilization within the past four months or had any history of recent illicit drug use. Tight security measures had been undertaken at the prison in the previous four months, to assure that no minor tranquilizers found their way illicitly to the blocks.

Three measures of hostility were taken. The first was the Hostility-Kindness scale of the Bipolar Psychological Inventory given routinely to all prisoners on their entry to the prison system. Representative questions of this instrument are shown in Appendix I. It has served the prison system well through the years as a basic guide to predicting hostility and aggressive activity among inmates although no test is perfect for all individuals. The second was a specially designed questionnaire produced in cooperation with the prison psychologists to measure hostility. Its reliability or validity cannot be vouched for since it was a one-time use, but its results are quite similar to the basic bipolar inventory. There was a significant, though small difference in the two groups in the pretest which was difficult to explain, but since they were similar in the two tests, and the differences in the posttest were not significant it was felt that the study was not jeopardized by this fact. A copy of this questionnaire is found in the Appendix.

The third measure was a report of all the detectable infractions of the rules from the medical technicians and correctional officers. These inmates were referred to the investigator for evaluation of the infraction to determine if it constituted rage reaction. These infractions included minor infractions of the rules of the prison, smuggling of the medication, psychological dependence on the drug as evidenced by requests for higher dosage or attempts to get the drug illicitly, confusion, and outright violence to himself or others. This last category included assault, attempted suicide, self-mutilation, and attempted murder.

Whereas the other two instruments were self-reports and depended on the patients' truthfulness in answering questions, this instrument was designed to be from direct observation. It was obviously not possible to observe and report every infraction of the rules since many are hidden in order to avoid punishment, but the technicians were instructed to refer every known incidence to the physician for evaluation. These were evaluated and recorded until the end of the study when the numbers of each kind of infraction were compared separately, the means and standard deviations were calculated and the two proportions calculated and compared by Z test and Chi square. Any paradoxical rage reaction as evidenced by violent and unusual outbursts of temper with or without injury was evaluated by the physician according to the offense, and recorded.

From our experience and the reported cases of paradoxical rage reactions in the literature (6), we had expected about a five percent rate for these rage reactions. This corresponded closely with our findings, but Valium® seemed to produce a significantly higher incidence of rage than Serax® even though the differences in hostility were not measurable by our instruments of measure.

All patients were continued on the drugs for one month except the nine who exhibited paradoxical rage reactions. The drug was discontinued on these nine immediately (Appendix) and the date of discontinuance recorded. Continuation of the drugs in these individuals might have been dangerous to themselves or others. During that time, all known infractions of the rules were recorded on the worksheet of all patients in the sample. The tests were given at two weeks in order to be uniform in the measurement of the effect of the drug, but the drugs were continued for a month to allow for any possible delayed paradoxical reaction. Minor infractions were defined as any infraction of the prison rules brought to the attention of medical technicians or prison guards and serious enough to require a write-up of the offense. Paradoxical rage reactions were defined as verbal or physical assault on an officer or other inmate,

4

Psychotropic Drug Research

attempted suicide, feelings of extreme hostility or anger, self-mutilation and attempted murder.

III. RESULTS

The average pre- and posttest scores on the scale of the Bipolar Psychological Inventory, Hostility-Kindness as shown in Table I reveals a small but significant difference between groups prior to the administration of the drugs but no significant difference after the administration of the drugs (pretest 5.62, 6.24. posttest 5.98, 6.52). The same small but significant difference appeared on the prison questionnaire in the pretest means but no significant difference in the posttest (Table II). (t Valium® = −1.319, Serax® = .4544). Table III separates paradoxical rage reaction from the other listed offenses according to definition and shows Valium® to have eight reactions or sixteen percent while Serax® showed only two percent. This was statistically significant (Z = −2.4460, p = .05). The Z test was used where the expected value fell below five in any cell. Otherwise the Chi square test was used.

TABLE I
Hostility scores of bipolar inventory.

Tranquilizer	Pretest		Posttest			
	Mean	S D	Mean	S D	t	Sig
Valium N = 50	5.62	1.58	5.98	1.39	−1.299	NS
Serax N = 50	6.24	1.21	6.52	1.57	.4762	NS

Drug comparison
pre-and postchange bipolar
inventory.

Valium		Serax			
Mean	S D	Mean	S D	t	Significance
+4.51	18.2	−.81	10.63	1.531	NS

SD = standard deviation

When all the other untoward reactions were grouped (Table IV), there was also a significant difference between Valium® and Serax® in their production of undesirable effects (Chi square = 4.32, p = .05). However, when all other infractions were separated (Table V), the difference in the two drugs was not significant. This may have

248

TABLE II
Hostility scores of prison
questionnaire.

Tranquilizer	Pretest		Posttest			
	Mean	S D	Mean	S D	t	Sig
Valium N = 50	57.26	16.94	61.36	13.65	−1.319	N S
Serax N = 50	64.62	11.86	63.40	14.58	.4544	N S

Drug comparison
pre-and postchange prison
questionnaire.

Valium		Serax			
Mean	S D	Mean	S D	t	Significance
4.26	20.50	−.72	11.92	1.47	N S

SD = Standard deviation.
Degrees of freedom = 98

TABLE III
Comparison of paradoxical
rage reactions.

	Valium		Serax			
	f	p	f	p	Z	SIG
Rage Reactions	8	.16	1	.02	−2.4460	.05

f = frequency;
p = proportion

TABLE IV
Comparison of all reactions
to the drugs.

	Valium	Serax	
Reaction	17	8	25
No reaction	33	42	75
Total	50	50	100 Subjects

Chi square analysis; Chi square = 4.32; degrees of freedom = 1; p = .05.

been at least partly due to dilution factors and small numbers exhibiting these reactions.

Psychotropic Drug Research

TABLE V
Comparison of all other
reactions

	Valium		Serax			
	f	p	f	p	Z	Sig
Minor infractions	0	.00	2	.04	−2.078	NS
Palming or smuggling	0	.00	3	.06	1.7586	NS
Psychological Dependence	6	.12	2	.04	−1.048	NS
Confusion or bizarre behavior	2	.04	0	.00	−1.428	NS

f = no. of reactions; p = proportion.

IV. DISCUSSION

Difficulties in the use of benzodiazepines in the control of anxiety in prisoners has renewed interest in finding a hostility tranquilizer. Research has been reviewed in finding the best use for Valium®, Librium®, Serax®, and Tranxene® in the attempt at modification of the behavior of prison inmates. The present literature is seriously lacking in prison studies. However, several articles are reviewed that describe experiences in which the use of various benzodiazepines are compared in individuals and groups, including private practices and psychiatric institutions. The general consensus is that most of the benzodiazepines must be used with caution in persons with real or latent hostility reactions, aggressive personalities, or who otherwise exhibit anti-social behavior.

However, if one of these drugs must be used it appears that Serax® (oxazepam) has certain advantages. The explanation for these advantages may lie in the fact that both Tranxene® and Serax® are metabolic breakdown products of Valium®. Since Valium® seems to be the greatest producer of euphoria, dependency and paradoxical rage reactions during the five to seven hours it remains in the system before being broken down into the less reactive products, Tranxene® and Serax®, in the liver, these reactions can be largely avoided by going directly to the final metabolic

250

Use and Misuse of Anxiolytics

products. The implications here are that Valium® should be used with extreme caution in prisoners or other aggressive populations. If a benzodiazepine is to be used, Serax®, being the final metabolic product should be used to minimize the chance of paradoxical reaction or interaction of metabolites. Future research will include better control of measurements and improved methods of observation in attempts to compare the minor tranquilizers with the major group such as Thorazine® or Stelazine® in the control of anxiety and hostility in prisoners.

V. SUMMARY

Past experiences with the benzodiazepine group of drugs in the population at the Utah State Prison are presented and indicate that the benefits derived from the administration of these drugs in prisoner control are nearly outweighed by the appearance of paradoxical rage reactions and increase in aggression, hostility, and dependence.

Serax® is suggested as a superior drug to Valium® for the purpose of anxiety control in hostile individuals if indeed a tranquilizer of this type is indicated.

REFERENCES

1. Barrett, J.E., and Di Mascio, A.: Comparative effects on anxiety of the "minor tranquilizers". *Dis. Nerv. Syst.*, 27:483-486, 1966.
2. Bobon, J., Collard, J., and Breulet, M.: Oxazepam or WY3498, a new preparation with tranquilizing and muscle relaxing properties and ambulatory treatment. *Acta. Neurol. Belg.* 65:327-334, 1967.
3. Gardos, G. et al: Differential actions of chlordiazepoxide and oxazepam in hostility. *Arch. Gen. Psychiatry* 18:757-760, 1968.
4. Hall, R., and Jeff, J.: Aberrant response to diazepam: A new syndrome. *Am. J. Psychiatry* 129:6 December, 1972.
5. Kochansky, G.E., Salzman, C., Shader, R.I., et al: The differential effects of oxazepam and chlordiazepoxide upon hostility in small group settings. *Am. J. Psychiatry* August 1975, pp. 861-863.
6. Lion, J.H., Hill, J., and Madden, D.: Lithium carbonate in the treatment of aggression. *Dis. Nerv. Syst.*, February 1975, pp. 97-98.
7. Madelina, J.C.: The therapeutic significance of the muscle relaxing psychotropic drugs in anxiety states. Psychiatry and Mental Health, *Fortaleza Cears*, July, 1965.
8. Salzman, C., et al: Is oxazepam associated with hostility? *Arch. Gen. Psychiatry* 31:401-405, 1974.
9. Warner, R.S.: Management of the office patient with anxiety and depression. *Psychosomatics* 6:347-351, 1965.

10. Westermeyer, J., and Walzer, V.: Sociopathy and drug use in a young psychiatric population. *Dis. Nerv. Syst.*, December 1975, pp. 673-677.
11. Zucker, H.S.: Letter to the Editor. N.Y. State J. Med., April 15, 1972, p. 974.

Prison Developed Questionnaire

Name _____ Date _____

Today I Have Been	None or Slight	Mild	Moderate	Quite	Much
Restless, on the go					
Afraid of things					
Concentration problems, easily distracted					
Anxious and worrying					
Nervous, fidgety					
Inattentive, daydreaming					
Short tempered					
Shy, sensitive					
Failing to finish things started					
Sad, depressed					
Stubborn, strong willed					
Dissatisfied with life					
Uncautious, dare-devilish					
Irritable					

253

Today I Have Been	None or Slight	Mild	Moderate	Quite	Much
Outgoing, friendly, enjoy company					
Impulsive, acting without thinking					
Sloppy, disorganized					
Moody, have ups and downs					
Feel angry					
Have friends, popular					
Well organized, tidy, neat					
Tend to be immature					
Feel guilty, regretful					
Lose control of myself					
Feel hassled, harried					
Tend to be or act irrational					
Unpopular with others					
Poorly coordinated					

254

Use and Misuse of Anxiolytics

Bipolar Psychological Inventory
Hostility–Kindness

Hostility Scale Questions:

I feel that most people would take advantage of you if you gave them the opportunity.

I often think it is better to take advantage of another person before they take advantage of you.

"An eye for an eye, a tooth for a tooth" is a good philosophy to live by.

There are a few people I would like to see worked over.

I wouldn't hesitate to step on people if it would benefit me.

I dislike many people.

It makes me feel better to tell someone off.

Hitting someone is hardly ever necessary.

I feel that fighting is no way for people to settle their differences.

Turning the other cheek is better than fighting.

I often tell others of my dislike for them.

I must admit that I usually laugh at the misfortunes of others.

I have been in my share of fights.

I've never gone out of my way to avoid a good fight.

I often get in fights or arguments.

I very seldom talk back to people when they give me orders.

I have seldom yelled at people throughout my life.

I very seldom threaten anyone with a physical attack.

I haven't been in a fight for years.

I usually do not get even with a guy who has hurt me.

APPENDIX I
Table of research results

Author	Type of Study	Type of Patient	No. of Pts	Drugs Compared	Results
Salzman	Review of lit.	Clinic or private	unknown	Valium, Librium, Serax	Hostility and rage uncommon in Serax
Galbor	Case control	Private practice	400	Serax	Minimal hostility or rage reactions
Bobon	Case history	Private practice	52	Serax	No hostility or rage
Madelina	Case control	Psychiatric clinic	41	Serax	No hostility or rage
Zucker	Cohort	Psychiatric clinic	400	Serax	4 possible reactions
Gardos	Controlled double-blind cohort study	Volunteer college students	45	Serax, Librium, placebo	Serax best hostility tranquilizer. Not effective in mild anxiety states.
DiMascio and Barrett	Cohort double-blind placebo controlled	Student volunteers	100	Librium, Serax	Serax better in controlling hostility
Kochansky	Cohort	Group therapy patients	30	Librium, Serax	Librium increased hostility. Serax decreased hostility

Lion	Case history	Private practice	2	Valium, Tranxene	Paradoxical rage reactions
Westermeyer	Cohort	Psychiatric in pts at U of M. (15 to 21 yrs)	100	Illicit drugs and alcohol	Strong correlation between drug use and sociopathy
Hale	Case history	Emergency room pts	6	Valium	Aberrant response to Valium

Psychotropic Drug Research

Analysis of Individual Rage Reactions

Mean scores on the Kindness-Hostility scale of the Bipolar Inventory for all inmates entering Utah State Prison 1974–1977.
Mean = 5176 Standard Deviation 3.55
Scores of inmates exhibiting rage reactions.

Number	Score	Percentile	Type of Reaction	Time
13254	7	70	Bizarre-aggressive irrational	5 days
13987	7	70	Felt violent, request be taken off	6 days
0838	8	79	Violent behavior, struck inmate	3 days
12793	1	3	Felt violent, meds stopped voluntarily	10 days
13176	9	85	Felt violent, verbal abuse, irrational	5 days
13750	4	39	Rage, violent struck several people	2 days
13573	9	85	Violent behavior, self injury (head)	7 days
14032	8	79	Irrational screaming struck an officer	3 days
13886	2	14	Rage, asked to be taken off medication	9 days

The mean of these scores is 5.1 and only one subject was more than one standard deviation from the mean. There was no significant difference in hostility scores between those who exhibited rage reactions and those who did not. There was a wide variation in percentiles of those who did exhibit rage by our definition but the rage reactions were not time or dose related. Number 14032 was on Serax® at the time of the reaction.

Index

Psychotropic Drug Research

oxotremorine, 68
oxytocin (OXT), 146-148

pain states, 150, 151, 153
Parkinsonism, 106, 107, 134, 138, 139
Prison Developed Questionnaire, 253, 254
prolactin (PRL), 119, 135
p-hydroxynorephedrine, 30
papaverine, 65, 66, 88, 89
paradoxical rage reactions, 243-245, 247, 249
pargyline, 33
pemoline, 78, 79, 82, 210
pentylenetetrazol, 78, 79
peptides, 117, 213
pharmaceutical needs, 51
pharmacological profile, 165
phenobarbital, 205
phenoxybenzamine, 211
phentolamine, 211
phenylephrine, 30, 31, 69
phenylhydantoin, 205
physostigmine, 81
pipradol, 78, 79
piracetam, 85, 86, 93
platelet MAO activity, 10, 13
  psychiatric disorders, 13, 14
  schizophrenia, 15-21
posterior pituitary hormones, 146
presbyophrenia, 80
primidone, 205, 207
progesterone, 212
propranolol, 211
psychotic episodes, 195
pyrithioxine, 91
pyritinol, 84

REM sleep, 77
RNA
  in memory, 81, 82
  receptor binding sites, 59
receptor subsensitivity modification (RSM), 105, 107, 112, 114
regional cerebral blood flow, 86-89
Renshaw cells, 213
reserpine, 32, 41, 43, 45
retinal system, 70

schizoaffective disorders, 7, 8
schizophrenia, 4, 6, 15, 18, 20, 43, 72, 107, 113, 132, 136, 142, 149, 151, 205
  platelet MAO activity, 13, 14, 16, 17
  propranolol, 211
scopolamine, 81
senescence, 51-53, 67, 71, 75
senile plaques, 83, 84, 92, 94
Serax® (see oxazepam)
serotonin, 34, 67, 208, 209
Sinemet®, 110
sleep rhythm, 76-79
sodium butabarbital, 77
soft neurological signs, 192, 235
somatotropin release inhibiting factor (SRIF), 117, 139
spiroperidol, 71
striatal dopamine system, 105, 106, 108, 109

tardive dyskinesia, 106, 107,

112, 113
temazepam, 77
testosterone, 212
thalamus, 213
threonyl-valyl-leucine, 155
thyroid stimulating hormone (TSH), 117, 119, 128-132, 135, 145
thyrotropin-releasing hormone (TRH), 117, 118, 120-135
Tranxene® (see clorazepate)
triazolam, 77
tricyanoaminopropene, 82
tricyclic antidepressants, 34, 36, 39, 41-43, 210
tubero-hypophysial system, 70
tyrosine hydroxylase, 42, 44, 59, 69

unipolar endogenous disorders, 8, 13
unipolar nonendogenous disorders, 8

VMA
  equation for D-type scores, 9
  excretion, 4, 8
Valium® (see diazepam)
vasopressin, 83, 146
vitamin E, 57, 58, 60, 72, 89

withdrawal dyskinesia, 106